THE
CHILDBEARING
DECISION

Published in cooperation with the
NATIONAL COUNCIL ON FAMILY RELATIONS

Series Editor: **John Scanzoni**
Family Research Center
University of North Carolina, Greensboro

Books appearing in New Perspectives on Family are either single or multiple-authored volumes or concisely edited books of original articles on focused topics within the broad field of marriage and family. Books can be reports of significant research, innovations in methodology, treatises on family theory, or syntheses of current knowledge in a subfield of the discipline. Each volume meets the highest academic standards and makes a substantial contribution to our knowledge of marriage and family.

Other volumes currently available from Sage and sponsored by NCFR:

THE VIOLENT HOME: A Study of Physical Aggression Between Husbands and Wives,
  Richard J. Gelles
ROLE STRUCTURE AND ANALYSIS OF THE FAMILY, *F. Ivan Nye*
SONS OR DAUGHTERS: A Cross-Cultural Survey of Parental Preferences,
  Nancy Williamson
CONFLICT AND POWER IN MARRIAGE: Expecting the First Child, *Ralph La Rossa*
THE AMERICAN FAMILY: A Demographic History, *Rudy Ray Seward*
THE SOCIAL WORLD OF OLD WOMEN: Management of Self-Identity,
  Sarah H. Matthews
FAMILIES AGAINST SOCIETY: A Study of Reactions to Children with Birth Defects,
  Rosalyn Benjamin Darling
ASSESSING MARRIAGE: New Behavioral Approaches, *Erik E. Filsinger and
  Robert A. Lewis, eds.*
SEX and PREGNANCY IN ADOLESCENCE, *Melvin Zelnik, John F. Kantner,
  and Kathleen Ford*

SINGLES: Myths and Realities, *Leonard Cargan and Matthew Melko*
THE CHILDBEARING DECISION: Fertility Attitudes and Behavior, *Greer Litton
  Fox, ed.*

THE CHILDBEARING DECISION

Fertility Attitudes and Behavior

Greer Litton Fox

Published in cooperation with
the National Council on Family Relations

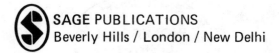

SAGE PUBLICATIONS
Beverly Hills / London / New Delhi

Copyright © 1982 by Sage Publications, Inc.

For information address:

SAGE Publications, Inc.
275 South Beverly Drive
Beverly Hills, California 90212

SAGE Publications India Pvt. Ltd.
C-236 Defence Colony
New Delhi 110 024, India

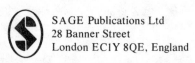

SAGE Publications Ltd
28 Banner Street
London EC1Y 8QE, England

Printed in the United States of America

Library of Congress Cataloging in Publication Data

Main entry under title:

The childbearing decision.

(New perspectives on family)
Published in cooperation with the National Council on Family Relations.
Includes bibliographies.
1. Birth control — United States. 2. Parents — United States — Attitudes. 3. Family Size — United States. 4. Communication in birth control. I. Fox, Greer Litton. II. National Council on Family Relations. III. Series.
HQ763.6.U5C48   304.6′66   82-3354
ISBN 0-8039-0136-4   AACR2
ISBN 0-8039-0137-2 (pbk.)

FIRST PRINTING

Contents

Series Editor's Foreword

While fertility control research in the United States spans several decades, during the past ten years we have experienced a rather remarkable convergence among numerous investigators regarding a potentially fruitful approach to understanding and predicting it. And in describing the decision-making approach to human fertility control, this volume represents virtually every major conceptual and methodological development in connection with it that has appeared in the literature. Fertility decision-making is an exceedingly complex phenomenon containing many facets, and at present there is no single demonstrably superior way to study it. This volume summarizes connections between decision-making and factors such as socialization, sex roles, work, motivational variables, and divorce. Researchers and practitioners alike will find that this book provides a solid base of information on which to build and extend their own future work. Professor Fox is to be congratulated for organizing and carefully shepherding such a rich and stimulating volume.

— John Scanzoni

Introduction

Greer Litton Fox

The substantive context for this book is formed by several remarkable changes over the past two decades in the sociology and social psychology of bearing children in this society. One of these changes is a widespread decline in fertility levels for the nation as a whole (Gibson, 1976). As Sweet (1974) documents in his recent analyses of this phenomenon, the fertility decline has characterized a broad range of social groups, including women at all socioeconomic and educational levels, racial identifications, and religious groups (see also Rindfuss and Sweet, 1978). The present low levels of fertility are the culmination of a broad-gauged and long-lasting fertility decline which followed the postwar peaks in levels of childbearing during the decade from the mid-1940s to the mid-1950s.

There is much evidence of change in couples' fertility patterns as well. Along with the steady increases in age at marriage and postponement of marriage into the mid-to-late twenties on the part of large proportions of young men and women (Glick and Norton, 1979), we find that today's young couples have longer marriage-to-first-birth intervals and longer second-birth intervals as well (Ford, 1981). This implies that they are not only more likely to be older parents than previous marital cohorts, but they may also be more mature during the marital period, when childbearing decisions are likely to be made. Today's young couples are also less likely to have third- and higher-order births (Ford, 1981), which suggests that despite later starts and longer birth intervals, they are likely to be younger when they cease bearing children.

[9]

Part of the change in fertility behavior shows up in changes in patterns of contraceptive use. Over the past two decades the use of contraceptives has become increasingly widespread (Westoff, 1976), and the major sociocultural differentials in use rates, such as religion, education, and economic status, have become attenuated (Mosher, 1981). Moreover, contraception has shifted from the less to the more reliable and effective methods. This implies that child number and spacing control is within reach and that family-planning decisions may be focused on whether and when to have a child within a more general decision context in which not to have children is the prevailing decision.

Alongside these shifts in childbearing behavior are shifts in the ideology of bearing children, as well. That there has been an increase in support for the option of childlessness is reflected in the birth expectations of young women; somewhat larger proportions of younger women expect to have one child or to remain child-free (U.S. Bureau of the Census, 1975). A different kind of shift is in attitudes toward the birthing process itself, as reflected in the movement toward the demedicalization and deinstitutionalization of the delivery, so that control over the process can be returned to the participants themselves. The development of outpatient birthing centers, the increase in the number of childbirth preparation courses offered both within and outside the formal medical delivery system, the interest in "natural" childbirth and breastfeeding, and the increase in the number of trained midwives are indicative of an ideological shift in our understanding of the social significance of bearing children. Yet another change is evident in the growth of positive attitudes toward the participation of the male partner prior to, during, and following childbirth in the care of the infant. Each of these changes in attitude and ideology is consistent with a loading of importance onto each child. That is, the scarcity of children may make them more precious. Thus, we might expect that conceptions and births alike will increasingly be intended and wanted — that they will be products of more considered, self-conscious, and concerted decision-making on the part of both partners.

In contradistinction to the preceding patterns are two other important trends in childbearing: the rise in the number of pregnancies and out-of-wedlock births among teenage women (Zelnik and Kantner, 1978), and the increase in the number of postmarital births among ever-married women (Rindfuss and Bumpass, 1977). In the study of teen childbearing the major decisions of interest are the decision to become sexually active, decisions about the use of contraception, and pregnancy resolution decisions. The latter two decision areas are also of primary interest in the study of postmarital fertility.

There is a long tradition of interest in the role of social and psychological factors in fertility research, and this volume lies squarely within that tradition. While the tradition has been eclipsed in recent years by a greater concern with economic models of fertility behavior, improvements in measurement technology, in modeling decision-making, and in complex analytic strategies have rekindled an interest in the role of motivational, psychological, and interpersonal interaction processes in fertility behavior. Many of the authors whose work is represented herein are actively working on the frontiers of such research.

Before turning to a chapter-by-chapter overview, a brief history of the development of the book is in order. The initial impetus came from Howard B. Gallas, a developmental psychologist with strong interests in psychological determinants of childbearing decision-making. After consultation with me and other sociologists, he established a working outline of this volume and invited a number of researchers from a broad spectrum of disciplinary approaches and perspectives to contribute chapters to this book. Although some were asked to concentrate on methodological stumbling blocks and solutions, others to report on innovative research designs in underexplored areas, and still others to review and reconceptualize certain segments of the fertility literature, the unifying theme for the work was our interest in exploring the antecedents, contexts, and processes of fertility decision-making from a variety of perspectives. After initiating the project, Gallas's interests shifted, and I was asked to take over the editorial role. While the present book departs somewhat from its original outline, the emphasis on an exploration of fertility decision-making from multidisciplinary perspectives remains intact, as the following overview of the contents shows.

In the first chapter Fox, Fox, and Frohardt-Lane propose a life-course model of the process of fertility socialization. They suggest that, for analytic purposes, the domain of fertility be subdivided into three sets of variables, according to their proximity to childbearing behaviors. Thus, "primary" foci would include measures of actual childbearing; "secondary" foci would include number and timing attitudes and values; and "tertiary" foci would include values, beliefs, and behavior regarding sex, family composition, sequencing, and the like. In their model they emphasize both macro-level societal variables and micro-level interaction contexts as loci for the development of fertility-related values and attitudes, which are reflected in and later affected by subsequent fertility behaviors. Their broad-gauged conceptual model provides a framework within which the remaining chapters in this volume can be placed. The second half of their chapter includes an empirical examination of the model, using data on the fertility attitudes of young teenage women as the focus of analysis. The authors not only find support for the overall model but are able to suggest several refinements.

In their chapter, "Sexual Decision-Making," Frank and Scanzoni develop a model of the dynamics involved in three areas of sexual decision-making: choice of sexual partner and participation in coitus, contraceptive use, and the expression of preferences for enhancing sexual satisfaction. Frank and Scanzoni suggest that sexual decisioning can be accounted for as a process that moves through the three evolutionary stages of exploration, expansion, and commitment. Within each stage the actual decision process is analyzed in terms of context, explicit and implicit interactive processes, and outcomes that either terminate the interaction sequence or cycle it into the next stage of decision-making. Thus the model synthesizes conceptual work in the area of the development of sexual relationships with work on generalized decision-making. Although in this chapter the authors apply their model to sexual behaviors they feel are most characteristic of young adults, they argue for its applicability to sexual interaction more generally.

Methodological problems in defining, measuring, and modeling the development and implementation of fertility decision-making at the *dyadic* level of analysis are considered in Beckman's chapter. In her analysis Beckman grapples with the difficulties posed by couple-level rather than individual-level responses, problems posed by our use of discrete rather than continuously distributed outcome variables, measurement error, and the difficulties of modeling complex, sequential, and reciprocal interactive processes. In the second part of her chapter Beckman provides an illustration of how such problems are encountered and can be dealt with in studying fertility decision-making, using data from her own research on couple decision-making. Beckman's discussion emphasizes the caution needed in utilizing multivariate techniques, such as regression, factor analyses, and LISREL, as applied to childbearing decision-making.

In contrast to the methodological orientation of Beckman, Rosen and Benson present a critical review of the corpus of work on fertility and family-planning decisions from the perspective of the male partner. They seek, in essence, what we can learn from the existing literature about the male partner's role in family size and child-spacing decisions, decisions about contraceptive use, and pregnancy resolution decision-making. They account for the paucity of information on male partners in terms of the difficulties of couple-based research, especially when the couple is in a temporary nonmarital union, and in terms of general cultural biases that define the childbearing domain as female. Rosen and Benson then review findings from their own research on the sources and nature of influence of the male partners on teenage women's pregnancy resolution decisions, and conclude with recommendations for continued research efforts with male partners.

In "Adolescent Contraceptive Use: The Impact of Family Support Systems," Herceg-Baron and Furstenberg consider a different source of influence on contraceptive and childbearing decisions, that is, the family. The authors consider whether, for adolescents, family members such as sisters or mothers may be important in influencing sexual, contraceptive, and childbearing decisions. After reviewing the available literature on this topic, they describe the preliminary outcomes of a research and demonstration project they designed. The purpose of their project was to assess the impact of systematic involvement of family members as part of a programmatic response to adolescent girls seeking contraceptive or pregnancy-planning assistance from Philadelphia-area family-planning clinics. Their early results suggest that increased family involvement is not necessarily associated with more effective contraceptive practice. An implicit result of their study is the reminder that intrafamilial and intergenerational influences on fertility-related attitudes and actions of teens are at least as complex phenomena as the couple-based decisioning processes analyzed in the preceding three chapters.

Campbell, Townes, and Beach look at motivational bases of childbearing decisions on the part of married couples. Their work thus falls squarely within the context of research on the psychological determinants of fertility. After reviewing this research, they apply a subjective expected utility decisioning model to data collected from some 200 married couples in the Seattle metropolitan area. They discuss measurement of couples' positive and negative utilities for childbearing, finding few differences by sex in motivational values for children. Moreover, they find a commonality across parity levels in the desire for close affiliation with the child as the major motivation for childbearing. At the same time, they find substantial differences by parity level across overall distributions of motivations and in total subjective expected utility scores. The authors conclude that it is possible to measure meaningfully personal motivations for childbearing and that tracing changes in such motivations during the period of family building provides clues for better understanding the process leading to differential levels of completed fertility per couple.

Whereas the Campbell et al. chapter examines childbearing motivations in terms of values attached to children, McGillicuddy-DeLisi and Sigel take a different tack in their chapter, "Family Constellations and Parental Beliefs." The authors argue that the investigation of parental beliefs about ideal family constellation, that is, family size and spacing of children, and about the impact of family constellation of the development of the child has become an increasingly important area of study in the examination of fertility decision-making. They present their research comparing views of parents of one-child families, of three-child families with short birth intervals, and of three-child families with longer birth intervals. While the authors are not willing to conclude that parental beliefs can predict to family constellation, they do find that parental views of the advantages and drawbacks of different family constellations appear to be linked to the actual number and spacing of children within their own families. Moreover, actual family constellations tended to reflect the parents' views of what is best for their child's social and personality development. They conclude that parental decisions about spacing and number of children are likely to be influenced by the parents' views of how family constellation affects children.

In "Early Mother-Child Interaction: Families with Only and Firstborn Children," Feiring and Lewis provide an implicit empirical examination of the expectation that parental fertility decisions may be influenced by parents' experiences with their firstborn children. The chapter presents results of the authors' analyses of mother-infant interaction during the first two years of the life of the child, comparing children who subsequently acquired a sibling with those who continued to be only children after 48 months. Among their findings are that only children as infants were fussier, less cognitively alert, and less sociable than the infants who later became firstborns. Moreover, mothers of only children were older at the birth of the child, desired fewer children, and had a more difficult childbearing experience than mothers who had subsequent children. The authors are not willing to say definitively that the observed differences in the infants, mothers, and their patterns of interaction are the causal factors in why some children gain siblings while others do not, but their findings suggest the fruitfulness of additional work in this area.

Sweet's chapter, "Work and Fertility," provides a broad overview of the conceptual and empirical work in this area, which has been a major focus of fertility analysis over the past decade or more. Sweet describes four different theoretical approaches that have been taken to the linkage between women's employment and fertility. These are the normative perspective, a sociological orientation that emphasizes the expectations for and sanctions attached to maternal versus worker roles for women; a time-allocation perspective, an economic orientation that analyzes fertility and work performance in terms of the relative utilities provided by each; a social-psychological career commitment or sex role socialization perspective; and a life-cycle or experiential perspective, deriving from social demography, which suggests that work orientation and fertility goals may shift as women move through the life cycle. Then, following a critique of the search for a single causal model of the work-fertility link, Sweet proposes three areas for future research: the processes through which age at marriage and age at first childbearing affect reproductive and work decisions; the impact of the "quality" of employment on a woman's reproductive and employment decisions; and, finally, the processes through which the economic conditions prior to and during the early years of marriage influence employment, marital, and reproductive decisions.

The continuation of high rates of marital dissolution and remarriage underscore the importance of understanding how patterns of marital behavior affect childbearing. In Chapter 10, Koo and Suchindran tackle the methodological problems of assessing the impact of marital discord, dissolution, and remarriage on fertility. First, they consider several general problems involved, such as the complexity of the relationships among the phenomena of interest, the likelihood that the nature of the interrelationships among the varibles changes over the course of the marriage, the possibility of sex-differentiated effects, and so on. Prior to suggesting specific approaches to dealing with each of these problems, the authors consider the strengths and limitations of retrospective, cross-sectional studies based on large probability samples as the most appropriate kind of data base for investigating the impact of marital quality and history in childbearing. Finally, the authors provide thorough discussions of a variety of approaches, accompanied by illustrations of their use, that will serve as a primer for those interested in research in this area.

Just as the increasing frequency of divorce and remarriage has necessitated the development of analytic approaches for measuring their relationship to childbearing, changes in the social and legal availability of pregnancy resolution alternatives call for an examination of the processes involved in the decision to terminate an elective pregnancy, to carry the child to term and rear the child on one's own, or to release him or her for adoption. Thus, in the final chapter, Rosen provides a critical review of the literature on pregnancy resolution decision-making. Rosen notes at the outset that much of the research in this area has focused not on the decisioning process but rather on the correlates of the decision outcomes. She characterizes the existing literature as having been dominated by three alternative value orientations that have colored the research designs and outcomes, including a deviance perspective, a feminist perspective, and a problem-solving perspective. She inventories the methodological shortcomings of the research, which she presents as both an impetus and an agenda for future work in this area.

As the preceding overview makes clear, the individual chapters vary greatly. Some provide descriptions of individual research efforts that highlight new or underresearched aspects of childbearing decision-making. Others are much broader in scope, with an emphasis on a critical synthesis and stocktaking of subsets of the fertility decision-making literature. Some authors were asked to concentrate on methodological problems and solutions; others were asked to work toward theory-building and overarching conceptualizations. Through the diversity of its chapters, the book as a whole provides many windows from which to gain an overall picture of the processes and factors involved in childbearing decisions.

REFERENCES

Ford, K. Socioeconomic differentials and trends in the timing of births. *Vital and Health Statistics* (Series 23, Data from the National Survey of Family Growth; No. 6. DHHS Publication [PHS] 81-1982), February 1981.

Gibson, C. The U.S. fertility decline, 1961-1975: The contribution of changes in marital status and marital fertility. *Family Planning Perspectives* 1976, 8 (September/October), 249-252.

Glick, P. C., and Norton, A. J. Marrying, divorcing, and living together in the U.S. today. *Population Bulletin*, 1979, 32 (5).

Mosher, W. D. Contraceptive utilization, United States, 1976. *Vital and Health Statistics* Series 23, Data from the National Survey of Family Growth; No. 7. DHHS Publication [PHS] 81-1983), March 1981.

Rindfuss, R. R., and Bumpass, L. L. Fertility during marital disruption. *Journal of Marriage and the Family,* 1977, 39, 517-528.

Rindfuss, R. R., and Sweet, J. A. The pervasiveness of postwar fertility trends in the United States. In K. A. Taeuber, L. L Bumpass, and J. A. Sweet (Eds), *Social Demography.* New York: Academic Press, 1978

Sweet, J. A. Differentials in the rate of fertility decline: 1960-1970. *Family Planning Perspectives,* 1974, 2 (Spring): 103-107.

U.S. Bureau of the Census, Fertility expectations of American women: June 1974. *Current Population Reports,* Series p-20, No. 277 (Spring): 103-107.

Westoff, C. F. Trends in contraceptive practice: 1965-1973. *Family Planning Perspectives,* 1976, 8 (2), 54-57.

Zelnik, M., and Kantner, J. F. Contraceptive patterns and premarital pregnancy among women aged 15-19 in 1976. *Family Planning Perspectives,* 1978, 10 (3), 135-142.

1

Fertility Socialization

THE DEVELOPMENT OF FERTILITY ATTITUDES AND BEHAVIOR

Greer Litton Fox, Bruce R. Fox,
and Katharine A. Frohardt-Lane

Compared with other substantive areas within the study of fertility behavior, the study of *socialization* for fertility is in its infancy. Throughout its short history, however, there have been a number of efforts to chronicle, and simultaneously to stimulate, the development of the research literature on fertility socialization (see, for example, the literature reviews of Russo and Brackbill, 1973; Gustavus, 1975; Philliber, 1980a, 1980b). In a series of recent papers, Philliber (1980a, 1980b) has articulated a conceptual framework for the analysis of population socialization, within which socialization for fertility behavior — the topic of this chapter — can be fitted. Philliber's contribution has been to inventory several dimensions relevant to population socialization, such as, the content of socialization, socializing agents, mechanisms, and timing. While this catalog is important at this stage as an organizational device, the framework itself provides little insight into the possible interconnections among the dimensions that constitute it.

In our review of the fertility socialization literature, we found evidence of a number of empirical regularities obtained by different authors using different methods to examine the reflection of parental fertility values and behavior in their children's fertility values and behavior. With regard to family size norms, for instance, the research to date has focused largely on documenting and then attempting to account for the intriguingly consistent, but consistently weak, positive correlation between completed family size in families of orientation and procreation. The search for an answer to the question of how it is within families that one generation comes to replicate the childbearing patterns of its immediate predecessor has uncovered related positive associations between parental family size and the offspring's ideals about family size (Gustavus and Nam, 1970; Johnson and Stokes, 1976; Simmons and Turner, 1976; McAllister et al., 1974; Coble et al., 1965; Thornton, 1980) and between parental ideals and child ideals relative to fertility (Thorton, 1980). Variables that have emerged as conditions on both the strength and shape of these relationships are child's birth order (Johnson and Stokes, 1976; McAllister et al., 1974), the quality of the parent-child relationship (Coble et al., 1965; Johnson and Stokes, 1976; Simmons and Turner, 1976), parental socioeconomic status (McAllister et al., 1976; Thornton, 1980), parental sex role attitudes and behaviors (Johnson and Stokes, 1976; Presser, 1974, 1978; Scanzoni, 1975; Simmons and Turner, 1976; McAlister et al., 1974; Thornton, 1980).

Desite the consistency across studies in terms of variables examined and relationships found, there has been little overall cumulation and few attempts to pull the research together into a coherent framework. Also, with only one or two exceptions, there seems to have been little effort by researchers in this area to ground their work in theory. The anticipation of some increment to an understanding of fertility behaviors has encouraged us to try to elaborate more fully a model of socialization. In so doing, we will accept the challenge inherent in Philliber's work (1980a, 1980b) to build upon her initial conceptual framework. Following the description of our proposed model, we will examine its utility in accounting for expressions of fertility ideals among a sample of urban teenage women.

FERTILITY AND SOCIALIZATION DOMAINS

Fertility

We start by asking what is meant by "fertility" within the context of "socialization of fertility." That is, what is the conceptual or theoretical domain of focus and what specific operationalizations can be suggested? Philliber (1980a) has suggested four general content areas: sexuality, contraceptive use, family formation, and family composition and function. While we agree that these four content areas are central to fertility, we think it useful to treat the domain of fertility through an ordering of foci based on the proximity of the sets of concepts to childbearing.

The *primary* items to be explained by a model of fertility are therefore those variables that best describe facets of actual childbearing. Thus, age of initiation of childbearing, total number of children born, and spacing of children or birth intervals would be the primary foci. These variables are operationalized in measures of actual fertility behaviors.

As *secondary* foci we suggest that attitudes toward, beliefs about, or preferences for age at first birth, number of children, and child spacing be considered. These would be operationalized as desires, intentions, or expectations. Indeed, for young women and men who have not begun childbearing behaviors, "fertility" can be measured only at the level of attitudes (that is, desires, intentions, and expectations). The virtue of distinguishing between fertility behaviors (primary foci) and fertility attitudes (secondary foci) is that the link between them can be taken as problematic.

As *tertiary* foci of fertility socialization, we would include those behaviors that are preconditions for fertility, namely exposure to intercourse and fertility regulation behaviors. Additionally, we would include the values, orientations, and knowledge surrounding human sexuality; fertility regulation attitudes, values, and knowledge; attitudes and values relative to marriage and family as contexts for childbearing; attitudes and values relative to family composition, including sex and sibling structure; and finally, values attached to children per se.

These three sets of foci include those variables that are properly explained within the context of fertility socialization, but they do not include the many additional variables that have impact on the fertility variables. For instance, lifestyle preferences are particularly relevant to fertility, but we feel these can best be treated as explanatory variables for fertility rather than as tertiary foci in models of fertility socialization. By lifestyle preferences, we have in mind sex role attitudes and values, constructions of male and female parent roles, work plans, and preferences for various work-family combinations and sequences (see Scanzoni and Fox, 1980, for an elaboration of sex roles as lifestyle preferences).

Several questions are raised by this formulation and need to be addressed. First, what are the temporal interrelationships among the various dependent-variable foci defined above? Clearly, a simple linear chain from antecedent lifestyle preferences through tertiary and secondary foci to actual fertility behaviors does little justice to the bits of empirical literature that are relevant to understanding the interrelationships among the variables. For example, the birth of the first child has enormous ramifications for lifestyle preferences and attitudes toward future childbearing among new parents (Russell, 1974; Hobbs and Cole, 1976), suggesting a complex web of reciprocal causation among these variables. Moreover, it appears that attitudes about childbearing and family size are learned very early; elementary-school-age children have been found to be able to articulate stable family size preferences in several studies (Frohardt-Lane et al., 1977; Gustavus, 1973; Gustavus and Nam, 1970). It is likely that these values were formed much earlier than, for example, lifestyle preferences attached to work roles versus family roles or work-family combinations (Scanzoni, 1975), which we think are not fully formed until late adolescence (and which even then are subject to change; see Scanzoni and Fox, 1980).

Further, it is probable that as part of learning about sexuality (including sex role learning) in infancy and very early childhood, children come to differentiate between men and women in terms of their ability to bear children, and thus to link the property of "womanness" to childbearing.[1] If sex role differentiation and the presumption of fertility behavior are learned simultaneously, then one cannot argue for the causal priorty of the development of sex role preferences over fertility attitudes. In sum, although we have ordered the foci of a model of socialization for fertility for analytic purposes, the order should not be presumed to be a temporal or causal ordering, even though in some instances the ordering may take on those properties.

A second question that can be raised is whether the process of socialization for fertility is a unitary one; that is, is the process the same for all fertility socialization outcomes? For example, are parental views about sexuality and contraception equally important for firstborns and later borns? Is quality of the parent-child relationship a factor only in the development of family size norms, or is it important in other transmissions as well? We will be able to address this issue specifically in a later part of the chapter by comparing the socialization process for ideal age at first birth with that for desired number of children, using data from a survey of teenage women. However, we can suggest here that it seems most reasonable to us to expect that the process is not unitary, in that fertility-relevant values and behaviors are learned and modified throughout the life cycle. Moreover, modes of learning and reasoning vary across different development stages. Brim (1966) argues, for instance, that adult socialization can be distinguished from socialization at earlier stages in the life cycle. Finally, the effectiveness of socialization agents may vary across time and from one topic to another. Parents, for example, may be more effective in transmitting family size norms and fertility values than in transmitting sexual standards (see Troll and Bengtson, 1979). In sum, there are reasons to expect that the process of socialization is variable, depending in part on the dependent measures one chooses to study.

A third question pertinent to our formulation of the dependent variables in a model of socialization for fertility is whether people form coherent life plans in which the order and timing of fertility events are carefully positioned along with other life events (such as education, marriage, career entry, and so forth) or whether such events are largely unplanned and thus independent of one another. For young women at least a contingency orientation to decision-making about future life events has been posited as replacing an earlier planful orientation, the contingency orientation becoming most pronounced as young women approach transition points (such as graduation from high school or college) during late adolescence and early adulthood (Angrist, 1969).[2] While some have suggested that the contingency orientation is less in evidence among maturing young women of the present decade (Scanzoni and Fox, 1980), we feel that the question should be treated as an open one. In any case, the possibility that persons may shift over time in their decision-making orientations to life events needs to be taken into account in fertility socialization models.

Socialization

What justification is there for looking at fertility behavior within a socialization framework? We think it might be useful to review briefly the particular contributions to understanding of *any* behavior, fertility in this instance, that can come out of a socialization perspective. The socialization perspective suggests that fertility behavior be viewed as the outcome of a *process* of socialization toward particular values influencing behavior. The central question then becomes, how and from what sources are fertility-related values transmitted, and how do they come to be received and incorporated into one's cognitive structure so that they form part of the core value matrix out of which one makes decisions or enacts preferences for behavior?

Different models of socialization, growing out of developmental psychology and sociology, suggest alternative but complementary emphases in answering this question. Let us consider them briefly. From developmental psychology both social learning theory and cognitive developmental models of socialization emphasize modeling, countermodeling, imitation, identification, and sanction-contingent learning as major processes through which children come to incorporate the values and beliefs of significant others. Cognitive developmental models also underline the stage-differentiated nature of socialization; that is, we can expect that fertility-relevant values are learned in different ways at different stages of development. Moreover, different socialization agents will have varying degrees of potency overtime — some receding, others gaining in importance — as the child's environment expands and as his or her capacity to engage the environment becomes more sophisticated.

From sociology the sybolic interaction perspective on socialization emphasizes the *social* nature of socialization by suggesting that the transmission of values and information occurs through interaction with significant others who provide models, standards for performance, and performance evaluation through encouragement or disapproval. Thus, it directs our attention toward the identification — in both social structural and personal relationship terms — of significant others as socialization agents and suggests that the nature of their relationship (positive or negative, affective or affectively neutral, symmetric or hierarchical, and so forth) may condition the socialization process. In addition, symbolic interactionism, through its focus on social *interaction,* draws attention to the *active* role of ego in one's own socialization in seeking information, initiating interactions, interpreting meanings, evaluating messages and performances, choosing values and behavior, enacting preferences, and deciding on actions. This orientation, which is also implicit in cognitive developmental approaches to socialization, is an important corrective to the view of persons as passive recipients of social transmissions entrapped in static socialization contexts, a view that all too often underlies deterministic models of socialization.

Having attempted to specify our starting points — that is, what kinds of variables might a model of socialization of fertility account for and what are the unique contributions of a socialization perspective to understanding fertility, we will proceed with a description of a model of fertility socialization. In so doing we will draw upon the research literature in this area to amplify our points and justify our reasoning.

A MODEL OF FERTILITY SOCIALIZATION

Components of the Model

There are five major clusters of variables that we hypothesize to be of importance in the process of fertility socialization: societal variables, family of origin variables, institutional socialization contexts, interpersonal socialization influences, and individual variables.[3] Because of space limitations we will simply list many of the proposed influences, concentrating the bulk of our attention on the family as a central socialization context and on family members as a significant socialization agents. We offer this model as a *preliminary* sketch of the process of socialization for fertility. We note that the specification of links among components within each cluster of the model and across clusters is incomplete and, in some instances, not even attempted. We expect that a fuller development of the model will be possible with further conceptual and empirical efforts; and we anticipate that the present model, though incomplete, can suggest some useful directions for much of that work. The model is presented schematically in Figure 1.1.

Societal Variables

Sociohistorical Contingencies. The initial set of variables in this cluster we call sociohistorical contingencies. Included are such factors as war, natural catastrophies, major economic shifts, and so forth. These are factors over which the individual has little or no control and to which he or she has only a limited set of possible behavioral responses. One of the responses to sociohistorical contingencies that individuals have traditionally employed is some alteration in their fertility behavior. It is for this reason that we include this variable cluster in our model.

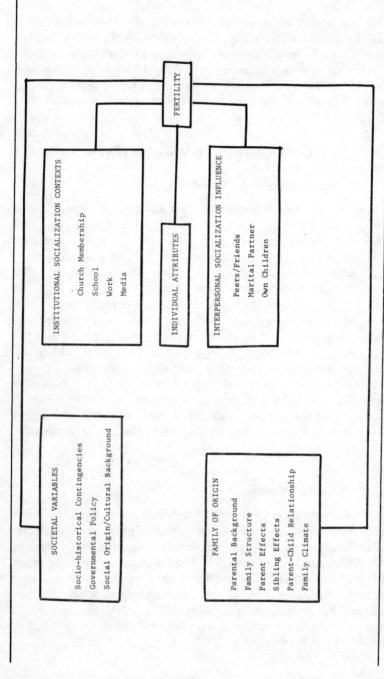

Figure 1.1 Conceptual Model of Socialization of Fertility Behavior

INSTITUTIONAL SOCIALIZATION CONTEXTS

Church Membership
School
Work
Media

INDIVIDUAL ATTRIBUTES

INTERPERSONAL SOCIALIZATION INFLUENCE

Peers/Friends
Marital Partner
Own Children

SOCIETAL VARIABLES

Socio-historical Contingencies
Governmental Policy
Social Origin/Cultural Background

FAMILY OF ORIGIN

Parental Background
Family Structure
Parent Effects
Sibling Effects
Parent-Child Relationship
Family Climate

FERTILITY

Governmental Policy. Governmental policies are the embodiment of societywide cultural values relative to fertility behavior. As such they are the backdrop of cultural uniformity against which subcultural values and individual preferences are formed and enacted. Included among the relevant policy variables here would be the restrictions on childbearing to certain populations (or the absence of restrictions). In general, the United States places no restrictions on childbearing; those who are able, may do so. From time to time, however, certain state legislatures have attempted to enact restrictions on childbearing, limiting the right to parenthood only to the "mentally fit" (thus excluding the developmentally disabled), to those women who have borne fewer than a certain number of children out of wedlock, and so forth. Another variable would be the degree of and conditions for availability of fertility regulation information, devices, or services (including contraception, abortion, and sterilization). The tax structure and supports for daycare vary in terms of their support for or penalties against families of different size and wage-earner combinations. Policies relative to welfare availability are relevant in that they express something of a society's valuation of quality of life for "any child." While some governmental policies have a clear and direct effect on fertility-related behavior (for example, the unavailability of medicaid abortions has a direct effect on childbearing in the absence of other means of payment), the effects of other policies are not nearly so clear (see Moore, 1980, for one attempt to assess the impact of policy variables on out-of-wedlock childbearing).

Social Origin/Cultural Background Variables. The third set of variables within this cluster comprises indicators of one's subcultural background or social origin, variables which, while measured at the individual level of analysis, take on their meaning only within the larger societal context. Included here are race, religious affiliation, nativity, ethnicity, urban-rural origins, regional background, and sex. Social origin variables are general descriptions or representations of probable socialization patterns. As such, they are expected to have little or no direct impact on fertility but rather to transmit the bulk of their impact through effects on other clusters of variables in the model. Indeed, the translation of social origin variables, such as race or ethnicity, into variables more proximate to fertility is one of the goals in understanding fertility behavior.

Family-of-Origin Variables

The family of origin is the primary context for socialization of the young child and continues to be significant in later years as well. There are several ways in which the family is expected to be involved in fertility socialization. First, we expect family members, especially parents to have direct effects on children's fertility values and behavior through intergenerational transmission of fertility values. Second, the parents' own fertility behavior can speak for itself, since it yields tangible, unequivocable, and objective evidence of parental actions. Parental behavior can be consistent with or counterposed against the parents' assessments and expressed evaluation of their own behavior (the latter is exemplified in the homily, "do as I say, not as I do"). The parents' behavior can be modeled or countermodeled by their children. A third mechanism through which families of origin impact children's behavior is through a filter or modifier effect on influences from external sources. Gagnon and Simon (1973) provide a nice description of this phenomenon as it operates in sexual socialization. Finally, through its social placement function the family determines (to a large degree for very young children and to a lesser degree for older children) an opportunity structure for exposure to socialization influences from outside the family.

Thus far, we have treated "family" as a global construct. It can usefully be disaggregated into the following smaller clusters of variables: *background, structure, parent effects, sibling effects, parent-child relationship,* and *climate.*

Parental Background. The background of the parent or parents can be assessed in terms of the social origin variables (above) and their location in social time (birth cohort, age) and social space (parents' work statuses, occupations, educational attainments, family social class, family income, and changes in these over time). As indicated earlier, several investigators have examined the association between parental measures on such variables and fertility values and behaviors of their children. In a recent review, Gecas (1979) pointed to the influence of parental socioeconomic status on a number of parenting behaviors. Thus, some of the association between family background and fertility ideals and behaviors may derive from the impact of family background on parenting styles.

Family Structure. This concept can be assessed in terms of family size, spacing and birth order of children, sex composition of siblings, sex/birth-order/spacing configurations and child density. Parental marital history and related measures such as continuity of parental dyad, sex of and number of household head(s), reconstitution of parental marital dyad, and presence of stepparent(s) would also be included as measures in family structure. As suggested earlier, at least some of these family structure variables, such as birth order, have been related to fertility values in offspring.

Parent Effects. In this variable set we include parents' own fertility-related attitudes, knowledge, and experience (including the premarital pregnancy experiences of parents); parents' expectations and aspirations for their children, the socioemotional tenor of the marriage as indicated by parental assessments of dyadic satisfaction and power and authority distributions, and parental assessments of satisfaction with parenting and family life. A number of investigators, cited earlier, have found that variables akin to "parental satisfaction with their life structure" condition the association between parent variables and the child's fertility behavior.

Sibling Effects. These would include the attitudes, knowlege, and experiences of siblings with regard to fertility. Although surprisingly little is known definitively about sibling influences (but see Kidwell, 1981; for a review of recent research, see Schvaneveldt and Ihinger, 1979), Spanier (1976) has suggested that siblings are of little importance to one another in sexual socialization during late adolescence. We would prefer to hold the question open and suggest that attention be directed toward investigating, for instance, the conditions under which one finds a "halo" effect resulting from a premarital pregnancy of a sibling as opposed to negative or countermodeling effects, or whether one finds positive correlations among adult siblings in terms of size of family of procreation. Further, whether siblings have effects on one another independent of their common inheritance of parental effects remains to be determined.

The Parent-Child Relationship. This concept can be assessed in terms of the degree of affect and the nature, extent, and content of interaction. Attention should also be directed toward the sex composition of the parent-child dyad; although the data are not altogether plentiful or clear, Troll and Bengtson (1979: 154) conclude that "gender differences are apparent in research on cross-generational family relationships."

Family Climate. In this variable set we would include such measures as family cohesion, the family's sense of group identity, family rituals and celebration, family religious practices, family sexual climate, and the like. We would not expect measures of concepts such as these to have direct effects on children's fertility values and behavior but rather to operate as mediator variables in the fertility transmission process, enhancing or dampening the effect of other family-of-origin variables.

Institutional Socialization Contexts

Church Membership. Association with and participation in a church community involves one in a socialization context in which specific sexual and fertility values and orientations are articulated.[4] The transmission of such values may occur through various sources, such as the church leaders, church-school teachers, the preaching or articulation of church doctrines, and church-related publications. Additionally, the church is often relied upon to reinforce parental value transmissions, in part by allowing parents to refer to a "higher" authority to legitimate their own precepts and teaching.

School. Another important socialization context is the school. In contrast to the church, which is likely to provide socialization content consistent with that received in the home, the school setting is the major source of exposure to alternative conceptualizations and orientations toward fertility-relevant values and behaviors. The school provides opportunities for experimentation with alternative attitudes and behaviors and for evaluation of one's performance in alternative roles. The school, as the major arena for heterosexual interaction, clearly structures one's opportunities for the initiation of heterosexual contacts.

The socialization agents within the school setting are varied. We would include teachers and their attitudes, values, and behaviors, the school curriculum, and the social and academic profile of the student body as a whole as well as its substructure and prestige hierarchies (the relative rankings of "academic" versus "vocational" tracks, athletes versus student elites, and so forth).

Otto (1979: 107-111) argues that the major effect of the school on marital timing comes through its impact on post-high school plans and aspirations for continued education or for immediate employment. He argues further that the channeling effect (into college-bound versus employment-bound futures) that schools can have on students is transmitted through the positive or negative evaluation of the student's performance in academic roles. The student who is rewarded by the school for scholastic performance, and who finds such rewards intrinsically meaningful, is more likely to continue to pursue his or her education than the student who receives few or no rewards for his or her efforts and for whom continuation in the system is costly. We think a similar argument could be made in terms of the impact of school on fertility values and behaviors.

Work. In the same way that the school setting (and the student role) is a major socialization structure for children, adolescents, and many young adults, the work setting (and the work role) is a socialization context for adults. Among the variables that could be included in this cluster are one's attachment to and performance in the work role, one's career aspirations and goals, the juxtaposition of one's work routine with that of one's partner or spouse, the intrusiveness of one's work role in nonwork domains, the actual and anticipated income from one's work, the demographic composition of the work force in one's immediate work setting, and the nature of one's relationship with work associates.

Media. The mass media (television, newspapers, magazines, radio, movies, records) must be considered socialization agents for fertility-related values and information in this society. Although their impact on family and child bearing values is relatively unexplored (although see LeMasters, 1974; Corder-Bolz and Cox, 1980), a few investigators have noted their influence in sexual socialization (Spanier, 1976; Weiss, 1974) and sex role stereotyping (see McGhee and Frueh, 1980; Weitzman, 1979).

Interpersonal Socialization Influence

Peers/Friends. As children mature, the friendship group takes on increasing importance as a context for, and individually as agents of, socialization. Indeed, Spanier (1976, 1977) argues that peers are of much greater significance in sexual socialization for high school and college youth than are parents or other adult figures (teachers, counselors, and the like). Presser (1978) found nonmodal dating frequency at age 16 to depress the age at first birth among young women whom she studied. We note that the "friends" of teenagers are likely to be made up almost exclusively of schoolmates, while for adults of childbearing age — 20 through 50 — the makeup of one's friendship network is more heterogeneous, with friends drawn from work associates, neighbors, church members, and so forth. Whether one's friends at these later ages continue to exert influence as socialization agents for fertility attitudes and behaviors is not known, but we suspect that they do so. We would argue that the following variables should be included in this cluster: the fertility-related attitudes, knowledge, and experiences of the friends; the friends' expectations for and evaluations of the individual; the frequency of contact with friends; and the intensity of affect and of the relationship and its extensiveness across behavioral domains.

Marital Partner. The marital partner, sex partner, or boy/girl friend is in one sense a special case of the friend/peer cluster above, and the variables indicated there would be pertinent in this cluster as well. We call special attention to marital partner, however, as a significant other in the process of fertility socialization, since his/her values, plans, and aspirations for the couple may be major considerations in an individual's own development of and shifts in preferences for sexual and fertility values and behavior (see Beckman, 1978, for example). In addition to assessing the partner's own values, knowledge, and experiences, one would need to assess his or her family origins as they relate to fertility outcomes.

Own Children. The response one has to the initial experiences of pregnancy, childbirth, and childrearing, as well as the nature of one's relationship with one's first child (or children), should be included in a model of fertility socialization. The effect of the first child on subsequent decision-making has been the subject of recent investigations (Hock et al., 1980; La Rossa, 1977; Miller and Sollie, 1980).

Individual Attributes

Among the attributes and characteristics of the individual that come into play in the development of fertility attitudes and behavior are his or her plans and aspirations for the future; his or her sex role preferences; his or her sexual standards and knowledge; the degree of heterosexual experience and evaluation or reaction to the experiences; personality traits and orientations; and birth-cohort membership. These individual variables are both summaries of the cumulation of socialization effects up to that point and variables that will shape future opportunities for socialization and thus future fertility behavior.

The Model as Process

The major components of the model have been introduced as clusters of cultural and subcultural background variables, family-of-origin influences, socialization contexts, significant others, and individual effects. Some comments about the timing of effects in the model are in order. Although there is a general developmental progression in terms of temporal order of effects through the life cycle, the order should not be treated as fixed. We emphasize that while socialization is a continuous process, it is not a unidirectional one; and because of the difficulty of establishing a temporal order among influences, it may not be best modeled as a causal progression. As suggested earlier, socialization contexts and socialization agents will be of varying importance as the individual moves through the life cycle. In addition, many of the predictor and outcome variables would lend themselves to measurement at several points in the individual's life cycle; we would expect their values and their level of association with one another to vary over the span of time covered by the model. Finally, the effects of these structures and variables are often continuously enacted rather than fully exhausted at a discrete point in time. For example, the mother's education is encountered as a variable at an early stage in the model we proposed, but we anticipate that its effect will in actuality be operative throughout the course of the child's interactions with his or her mother over the life cycle.

As for the operation of the model as a socialization process whose end products are some levels of fertility attitudes (the secondary foci) and behavior (the primary foci), we suggest that the initial influences toward fertility values to which a child is exposed are largely determined by his or her social origins and family background. These influence both the content and the contexts of socialization, in which parental attitudes and behavior are inferred and observed, modeled, imitated, reproduced in the child's early verbalizations and behaviors and either rewarded or extinguished.

As the child's effective environment expands, parental values and beliefs can be reiterated in other socialization settings by other socializing agents, thereby serving to reinforce the initial transmissions from parents. This is similar to the important "redundant socialization" effects discussed by Lamb (1978) and the "congruence" across socialization fields discussed by Bronfenbrenner (1970). Alternatively, socialization content at variance with that received from parents or other early socializers may be encountered by the child. This is more likely to be the case in the more elaborated or heterogeneous environments to which the child is increasingly exposed (and indeed may actively seek) as he or she matures.

We suggest that children (and adults as well) continuously evaluate the valuational and informational inputs they receive; make choices among alternative values and behaviors; try out those choices; and adjust them, discard them, or seek out new information from which to craft still other sets of values and behaviors, according to the responses (positive or negative) of the significant others who staff the salient socialization contexts that are operative at various points throughout the life cycle. The choice or preference for one set of values and behaviors rather than another reflects one's assessment of the relative balance of social and psychic costs and rewards that accompany the enactment of those behaviors and values (Scanzoni and Fox, 1980). But these can change over time. That is, as the assessment of the rewards and costs of one set of fertility values and behaviors changes over time, some shift can be expected in the individual's values and behavior. It is in this way that the model can allow for the socialization process to be portrayed as a continuous one, relevant to adult socialization as well as to preadult socialization for fertility.

APPLICATION OF THE MODEL

As an illustration of the ability of the model to provide a meaningful framework for understanding socialization for fertility, we will apply the model to data from the Mother-Daughter Communication re Sexuality Project,[5] an interview study of girls aged 14 to 16 and their mothers. While particular emphasis is given to family-of-origin variables and individual attributes, data are available on at least one variable from each of the major independent variable sets in the model. Two fertility-related attitudes of the teenage girls, their desired age at birth of their first child and the number of children they intend to have, are available for use as dependent variables.

In addition to considering the question of the applicability of the model as a whole, we also consider three questions that explore different aspects of the model. First, within groups with different social origin/cultural backgrounds, is the process of socialization the same? More specifically, is the process of socialization to these two fertility attitudes different for black and white teens? We already know that actual fertility differs for these two groups. Second, can one set of variables, namely the family-of-origin variables — particularly as related to the mother — be shown to affect fertility? More specifically, are mothers of teenage girls important agents of socialization in the development of the daughter's fertility attitudes, and can some specific sources of the mother's influence be identified? (The latter half of this question is dealt with in detail by Fox et al., 1981.) Third, if one chooses two different fertility variables, will the sources of influence be similar or will they differ?

Methods

Data Base. The data are drawn from a clustered, stratified sample of high school students enrolled in the public school system of a large central city. The 449 girls and their mothers who volunteered for the study were interviewed in separate but simultaneous face-to-face interviews, during which demographic, attitudinal, and behavioral information was obtained.

The sample includes persons from a broad spectrum of racial and socioeconomic backgrounds. Of the sample, 56 percent were black; 44 percent were white. Just under half (48 percent) of the daughters had lived continuously in maritally intact homes, while the remainder had experienced disrupted parental marital histories. Median family income in 1978 was $19,126; total family income for approximately 20 percent of the sample was less than $9,000, while for another 18 percent it was $30,000 or more. Just over half of the mothers (53 percent) were employed outside the home. One-fourth of the mothers had not completed high school, while one-third of them had had some postsecondary training. Nearly all of the daughters were 14 or 15 years old when interviewed, and at that time two-thirds of them were coitally inexperienced. (A more complete description of the study design and sampling procedures is contained in Fox and Inazu, 1980.)

Dependent Variables. The dependent variables chosen for study are the preferences of the teenage girls for two of the primary fertility variables: age of initiation of childbearing and total number of children born. As such, these attitudes/preferences are identified in the model as secondary foci of fertility variables. Since these teenagers had not yet begun bearing children, their actual fertility behavior could not be studied.

Desired age at birth of first child was ascertained by asking daughters to indicate their preferences on a time line. Nearly all gave ages between 20 and 30; there was some concentration at age 25, which was chosen by 20 percent of the sample. Intended number of children was assessed by asking how many children of their own they intended to have. A normative preference pattern was apparent, in that 43 percent of the daughters intended to have two children and 24 percent intended to have three children. Forty-one girls (9 percent) intended to remain child-free.[6]

Independent Variables. The Mother-Daughter Communication Project focused on determining the effect of the mother and the mother-daughter relationship on the daughter's attitudes and behaviors. Thus, in the present analysis of fertility socialization, parental effects, as represented by the mother-daughter relationship measures, are particularly well tapped. In addition, the survey contained data on individual attributes of the daughter that potentially are related to fertility attitudes. The independent variables were selected from the variables available in the survey data to represent each of the variable sets in the conceptual model. The correspondence between the independent variables used in the analysis and variables in the conceptual model is shown in Table 1.1.

Of the *societal variables* set, one variable, race, is included in the analysis. Since appreciable differences in socialization by race were expected, race is taken into account in the analysis through separate analyses for black and white daughters. For the purpose of this

TABLE 1.1   Correspondence between Variables in Conceptual Model of Fertility Socialization and Variables in Analysis

Variables in Conceptual Model	*Variables in Analysis*
Societal Variables	
Sociohistorical contingencies	
Governmental policy	
Social origin/cultural background	Race
Family-of-Origin Variables	Family Characteristics
	Relative family income (N)
Parental background — — — — — —	Mother's education (A)
	Mother's year of birth (N)
	Family size (A, N)
	Sex of household head[a] (A)
Family structure — — — — —	Cohabitation[b] (N)
	Daughter's birth order[c] (A)
Sibling effects — — — — — —	Number of pregnant sisters (N)
Family climate — — — — — —	Family religious practices (A)

TABLE 1.1 (Continued)

Variables in Conceptual Model	*Variables in Analysis*
Parent effects — — — — — —	Mother's Attitudes Sex role ideology[d] (A, N) Sexual knowledge[e] (A) Desired age for daugher's first birth (A, N) Desired age for daughter's first job (N) Sexual Satisfaction[f] (A) Educational aspirations for daughter (A)
Parent-child relationship	Mother-Daughter Relationship Relationship quality[g] (A, N) Preteen sex talks[h] (A) Daughter wants to be like mother (N) Daughter accepts mother's aspirations (N)

Institutional socialization contexts
  Church membership
  School— — — — — — — —
  Work
  Media
	Daughter's Current Situation
	  Grades (A)
	  Attends technical high school (A, N)
	  Normative dating frequency[i] (A, N)
	  Grade in school (A)

Interpersonal socialization influence
  Peers/friends – — — — — — —
  Marital partner
  Own children
	Daughter's Sexual Profile
	  Sexual knowledge[e] (A, N)
	  Sexual status[j] (A)
	  Permissiveness attitudes (A, N)

Individual attributes— — — — —	Daughter's Attitudes
	  Sex role ideology[d] (A, N)
	  Educational aspirations (A)
	  Desired age at first job (A)
	  Desired age at marriage (N)
	  Proper sex role behavior[d] (N)

a. 1 = female; 2 = other.
b. 1 = mother has not cohabited in daughter's life; 2 = mother has cohabited.
c. 0 = daughter is not oldest daughter; 1 = daughter is oldest daughter.
d. Higher scores = more modern attitudes.
e. Higher scores = greater knowledge.
f. 1 = high satisfaction; 3 = dissatisfaction.
g. Higher scores = more favorable assessment of relationship.
h. Number of sex-related topics discussed.
i. 1 = goes out on 2 dates per week; 2 = goes out on more or less than 2 dates per week.
j. 1 = virgin; 2 = nonvirgin.

A = included as predictor in analyses of desired age at first birth.
N = included as predictor in analyses of intended number of children.

analysis, the *family-of-origin* variables have been grouped into three sets: (1) family characteristics, which contains nine variables and represents parental background, family structure, sibling effects, and family climate; (2) mother's attitudes, which contains six variables and represents parental effects; and (3) mother-daughter relationship, which contains four variables and represents parent-child relationship.

Of the four *institutional socialization contexts* outlined in the model, two variables represent the school context. Data were not available to represent church membership, work, or the media. Two variables represent the peers/friends subset of the *interpersonal socialization influences*. Influences from marital partner and own children are not relevant to a sample of young teenagers. These four variables were grouped together in a set called "daughter's current situation." The set of *individual attributes* in the model is represented in the analysis by two sets of variables: daughter's sexual profile and daughter's attitudes.[7] The independent variables are thus grouped into six sets of variables that correspond to, but are not identical with, the variable sets in the conceptual model.

Method of Analysis

There were three steps to the analysis. In both the first and the second steps, each of the six sets of independent variables was regressed on the two dependent variables, using forward stepwise multiple regression analysis. For each independent variable set, three regressions were run, one for the total sample of 449 girls and one for each of the races separately.

The first step in the analysis was used to reduce the pool of independent variables. For each dependent variable, the forward stepwise multiple regressional analyses for blacks, whites, and total sample were compared. Variables that provided the best single set of predictors across all three sample groups were retained for the second analysis.

The second step of the analysis was designed to determine the contribution to explained variance in the dependent variables of each of the six sets of variables, and, within sets, the relative contribution of each separate independent variable. (Details of this analysis are presented in Fox et al., 1981.)

In the final step of the analysis, all six variable sets were entered into a multiple regression analysis, stepwise by sets, to determine the extent to which each set added to the variance explained by other sets. For this step, the three sets of variables based on the daughter (daughter's current situation, daughter's sexual profile, and daughter's attitudes) were combined, since none of the three sets was clearly antecedent to any of the other two sets.

Results

As can be seen in Table 1.1, the first step yielded two different lists of predictor variables to be used in later steps in the analysis. Although we required the same set of variables be retained for the two dependent variables. As a result, the overlap in the important predictors of the two dependent variables is far from complete. An inspection of the variables retained suggests that the specific items that influence fertility attitudes are, in this case, different for the different fertility attitudes. Thus, the daughter's desired age at birth of her first child and her intended number of children apparently result from different specific sources of influence.

Desired Age at Birth of First Child. The results of the second analysis are summarized in Table 1.2. (Detailed results, in which specific variables are discussed, are contained in Fox et al., 1981.) Table 1.2 shows that for the first dependent variable, desired age at birth of first child, each of the six sets of variables by itself accounts for a limited but significant portion of the total variance for the total sample and for blacks and whites separately. This provides support for the inclusion of each of the sets in the general model, at least insofar as the data were available to permit representation of the sets in the analysis. Since each of the six sets of predictors is significant for both racial groups, we can conclude that the general model identifies significant sources of socialization for both black and white daughters.

On the other hand, there are major differences by race. As shown in Table 1.2, the R^2 for the family characteristics set is higher within racial groups than for the total sample. This happens because three of the five variables within the family characteristics set have different directions of effect by race (details not shown). For the other five sets of variables, the portion of variance explained is greater for whites than blacks, particularly for the variable set "daughter's attitudes." The difference by race might be due to the use of items of more importance in the socialization of this fertility attitude for white girls or possibly to better measurement among this white subgroup.

TABLE 1.2 MRA of Daughter's Desired Age at Birth of First Child and Intended Number of Children: Total Variance Accounted for by Variable Set

| | Desired Age at Birth of First Child R^2 | | | Intended Number of Children R^2 | | |
	Total Sample	Black	White	Total Sample	Black	White
	(N = 449)	(N = 253)	(N = 196)	(N = 449)	(N = 253)	(N = 196)
Family Characteristics	.043*	.075*	.073*	.046*	.033	.089*
Mother's Attitudes	.072*	.070*	.115*	.037*	.031	.082*
Mother-Daughter Relationship	.050*	.053*	.062*	.017	.021	.023
Daughter Variables	.152*	.122*	.234*	.060*	.101*	.064
Daughter's current situation	.072*	.068*	.092*	.008	.017	.005
Daughter's sexual profile	.074*	.070*	.088*	.010	.043*	.030
Daughter's attitudes	.100*	.060*	.183*	.041*	.052*	.058*

*p < .05

Intended Number of Children. Prediction of intended number of children with the sets of variables included in this study was poorer than prediction of desired age at the birth of the first child. This may be partially a result of the comparative lack of variance in number of children desired, making it more difficult to predict what variance there was in the responses.

For the total sample, only three of the six variable sets accounted for statistically significant amount of variance as shown in Table 1.2. These were family characteristics, mother's attitudes, and daughter's attitudes. When the three daughter variable sets are combined in order to compare with the results of the cumulative analysis that follows, this set also accounts for a significant amount of variance. Two of the three sets of variables, which as a whole were not significant predictors of intended number of children, contain one variable that by itself is significant. Relationship quality within the mother-daughter relationship set and permissiveness attitudes within the daughter's sexual profile set are both significantly correlated with intended number of children for the total sample ($r = .10$, $p < .05$).

Only two variable sets emerged as significant predictors of family size intentions among the black daughters: daughter's sexual profile (due primarily to the variable permissiveness attitudes) and daughter's attitudes (due primarily to the girl's desired age at marriage). It is notable that for black daughters none of the indicators of family characteristics, maternal attitudes and relationships, or the daughter's academic and social situation was significant in the explanation of intended family size.

By way of contrast, for white daughters the family characteristics set and the mother's attitudes set each account for over 8 percent of the variance in family size attitudes among these daughters. In addition for the white daughters, as was the case for black daughters, the variable set daughter's attitudes accounted for a significant proportion of the variance.

The Cumulative Model. Thus far, we have looked at different components of the model, but we have not looked at it cumulatively. This is done in Table 1.3, which presents results from a stepwise forward regression analysis in which the variable sets were entered one at a time in what we felt to be a reasonable approximation of a temporal order. That is, the variables within the family characteristics set were entered first and allowed to account for as much of the variance in the dependent variables as possible. Then, the mother's

TABLE 1.3 MRA of Daughter's Desired Age at Birth of First Child and Intended Number of Children: Total Variance and Increase in Variance by Cumulation of Variable Sets

	Total Sample (N = 449)		Black (N = 253)		White (N = 196)	
	R^2	R^2 Inc.	R^2	R^2 Inc.	R^2	R^2 Inc.
Desired Age at Birth of First Child						
Family Characteristics (5 variables)	.043*	.043*	.075*	.075*	.073*	.073*
plus Mother's Attitudes (5 variables)	.088*	.045*	.121*	.046*	.144*	.071*
plus Mother-Daughter Relationship (2 variables)	.106*	.018*	.137*	.016	.167*	.022
plus Daughter Variables (10 variables)	.198*	.092*	.219*	.083*	.280*	.113*
Intended Number of Children						
Family Characteristics (5 variables)	.046*	.046*	.033	.033	.089*	.089*
plus Mother's Attitudes (3 variables)	.068*	.022*	.048	.015	.157*	.068*
plus Mother-Daughter Relationship (3 variables)	.087*	.019*	.071	.023	.171*	.014
plus Daughter Variables (7 variables)	.135*	.048*	.168*	.096*	.202*	.031

*p < .05

attitudes set was entered and allowed to account for unexplained variance in the dependent variables. The mother-daughter relationship set was entered next and it, too, was allowed to account for unexplained variance. The last three variable sets, all pertaining to the daughter, were entered into the regression simultaneously, since we felt there was no way to argue for the temporal priority among the three sets.

For the total sample and for both dependent variables, each set of predictors adds significantly to the explanation of the two fertility attitudes, lending strong support to the overall model. This can be seen in Table 1.3 in the column giving the R^2 increase for the total sample. Thus, family characteristics, mother's attitudes, mother-daughter relationship, and the combination of daughter's current situation, sexual profile, and attitudes each contribute to an understanding of the daughter's fertility attitudes.

As a whole, the variables used in the model of socialization for desired age at birth of first child account for almost 20 percent of the variance of this variable, while those variables in the model of socialization for intended number of children account for 13.5 percent of the variance in this variable. When the analyses are performed separately by race, the amount of variance explained increases, again suggesting the importance of considering these racial groups separately.

The analysis for desired age at birth of the first child reveals that for both black and white daughters the mother-daughter relationship variable set does not add significantly to the variance accounted for, once the antecedent variable sets have been taken into account. The R^2 increase is .016 and .022 for blacks and whites respectively, while the R^2 for these sets taken alone from Table 1.2 are .053 and .062. This suggests that the direct effect of these variables is partially accounted for by family characteristics and mother's attitudes.

Discussion

What answers have been found to the questions that we wanted to address in this analysis? First, our particular operationalization of the theoretical model outlined in the first section of this chapter received empirical support, especially in the explanation of daughter's desired age at birth of first child, indicated by the overall portions of variance explained in the outcome measures by the variable sets separately (Table 1.2) and by the model as a whole (Table 1.3). Adding to our confidence that the model of fertility socialization outline earlier has some explanatory utility is the fact that, for the sample as a whole, each of the components of the modes that we had hypothesized to be of importance in the determination of fertility-related attitudes did, in fact, contribute significantly to the explanations of both of the dependent measures (Table 1.3).

Second, we were interested in whether there might be evidence that the process of fertility socialization operated differently by race. The answer appears to be yes, since not only were different predictor variables significant for blacks and whites, but for a number of variables the direction of the impact on the dependent variables was reversed for the two races.

A third question concerned the role of the mother as an agent of fertility socialization for her daughter. For this question the results are harder to summarize. From the data presented it appears that in white families the mother's attitudes on a variety of lifestyle topics do influence her daughter's fertility timing and number values. In black families, the mother's attitudes are influential in terms of the daughter's timing values but not her intended family size. Whatever the source of the mother's influence as a socialization agent, it appears not to hinge importantly on our measures of the mother-daughter relationship (that is, the daughter's assessment of the quality of the relationship with her mother, the daughter's acceptance of the mother as a role model, the daughter's wanting to live up to her mother's expectations, and mother-daughter sexual communications prior to puberty). As was shown in Table 1.3, these variables add little more to the explanation of the daughter's fertility attitudes beyond the contributions of family background and maternal attitude measures. Mothers appear to influence their daughters more by who they are, so to speak, than by what they do directly with their daughters. Another way of stating this is that these data suggest that the mother's attitudes and value positions are transmitted to their daughters regardless of the daughters' assessments of their mothers and of their relationships with them.

Finally, we were interested in whether the same variables would be equally important in the predictions of the two dependent variables in our analysis. Clearly, here the answer is no. This was evident not only in the preliminary analysis but emerges from the analyses in Tables 1.2 and 1.3 as well. Further, the sharpest contrast between the racial subgroups is found here. For the black daughters in this study, attitudes toward desired timing of first birth were a function of a broad spectrum of variables, including distal background measures as well as the daughter's current attitudes and actions, whereas their attitudes about number of children were not significantly influenced by anything other than the "daughter" variables. For black daughters it may be that relative to the desired age for initiation of childbearing, number of children is viewed as the more flexible aspect of fertility; thus it would be more responsive to contemporaneous contextual contingencies (such as are indicated in the daughter variable set) and less fixed by background characteristics inherited along with one's family of origin.[8]

For the white daughters, the major difference in the socialization process for the two fertility attitudes hinges on the relative importance of the daughter variables. These variables were the most important predictors of timing attitudes, which is consistent with the "contingency orientation" to decision-making about life events, discussed earlier in the chapter. The same variables, on the other hand, were relatively unimportant in predicting their attitudes about intended family size, which, for white girls, appear to be a product of earlier socialization within the family and relatively untouched by potential sources of influence in the daughter's teenage world.

CONCLUSION

In this chapter we have sketched a broad model for the process of socialization for fertility behavior in order to provide an overarching conceptual framework within which the existing research literature in this area might be fitted and to provide a conceptual base on which new research efforts might be built. The model suggests that socialization for fertility is a long-term and continuously unfolding process, with influences stemming from a multiplicity of sources that shift in relative importance over the life cycle.

We offered an initial examination of the model, emphasizing certain elements of the model and omitting others, in accordance with the characteristics of our data set on mothers and teenage daughters. From the analyses performed, we conclude that socialization for fertility behavior is a unitary process only in the abstract, such as at the level of our overall model. When one is able to look more closely and comparatively at different outcome measures or at population subgroups, as we did, one finds a rich complexity of patterns operative in the determination of fertility attitudes and behavior. It is that complexity within the context of a simpler, more abstract, and over-arching model that will require further investigation before we can speak truly of a theory of fertility socialization.

NOTES

1. If , as we suspect, "childbearing" and "woman" become defined interchange-ably in the minds of children, then it would appear that children at very young ages come to hold pronatalist values. Girl children in particular would develop very early an expectation for their own future childbearing. We suggest further that the de-velopment of preferences for childlessness occurs through the process of *unlearning* earlier cognitions, as well as through a process of incorporation of *new* attitudes about childlessness. Our conjecture is given some support by the findings on volun-tary childlessness by Veevers (1973), Houseknecht (1979), and others that the deci-sion to remain childless is for most women a decision reached during adulthood rather than during childhood or adolescence (see Houseknecht, forthcoming).

2. Angrist (1969) suggests that the major contingency in the lives of young women is their unknown but anticipated future husband. Without knowing something of his identity, young women find it difficult to commit themselves to career choices, to pursue long-term career training, and, perhaps most tellingly, to believe that they can enact or implement with any degree of certainty the choices they might have made.

3. In his review of the literature on antecedents and consequences of marital timing decisions, Otto (1979) proposes a life-course model in which the antecedents of marital timing are categorized into the following sets of influences: social origins, socialization and significant-other influences, personality effects, contingencies, and post-high school plans and aspirations.

4. We are using "church" to refer to all religious denominations and divisions.

5. The Mother-Daughter Communication re Sexuality Project was conducted in 1977-1980 in Detroit, Michigan, under Grant HD11224 from the Center for Popula-tion Research at the National Institutes for Child Health and Human Development, with G.L. Fox as Principal Investigator.

6. Even though their intention was to remain child-free, all gave a desired age at birth of first child, perhaps because the time-line format did not provide for a no-child response. The girls may have felt that a response to this item was mandatory. To counter the possible error in the data on desired age at birth of first child, all regressions were run with and without the 41 cases. Difference in the results were quite small, so the analyses presented are based on the entire sample.

7. Daughter's desired age at marriage was excluded as a predictor for daughter's desired age at birth of first child, since they were both obtained from the same time line and their high correlation (r= .63) was therefore partially artifactual.

8. This analysis further suggests that models explaining the inverse relationship between socioeconomec status and family size norms in terms of the inheritance of tastes for "expensive" versus "cheap" children would not be appropriate for the black daughters but would be appropriate for the white daughters in our sample.

REFERENCES

Angrist, S. S. The study of sex roles. *Journal of Social Issues,* 1969, 25, 215-231.

Beckman, L. Couples' decision-making processes regarding fertility. In K. E. Taeuber, L. L. Bumpass, and J. A. Sweet (Eds.), *Social Demography.* New York: Acedemic Press, 1978.

Brim, O. G., Jr. Socialization through the life cycle. In O. G. Brim, Jr., and S. Wheeler (Eds.), *Socialization after childhood.* New York: Wiley, 1966.

Bronfenbrenner, U. *Two worlds of childhood: U.S. and U.S.S.R.* New York: Russel Sage, 1970.

Coble, J. M., Duncan, O. D., Freedman, R., and Slesinger, D. P. Marital fertility and size of family orientation. *Demography,* 1965, 2, 508-515.

Corder-Bolz, C., and Cox, C. *Impact of television upon adolescent girls' sexual attitudes and behavior.* Paper presented at the American Psychological Association Meetings, Montreal, Canada, September 2, 1980.

Fox, B. R., Frohardt-Lane, K. A., and Fox, G. L. Do as I say or do as I do: The transmission of fertility attitudes from mother to daughter. Family Research Center Working Paper M D-1 Wayne State University, 1981. (Available from authors on request.)

Fox, G. L., and Inazu, J. K. Patterns and outcomes of mother-daughter communication about sexuality. *Journal of Social Issues,* 1980, 36, 7-29.

Forhardt-Lane, K. A., Landis, J. R., and Bruvold, W. H. A new technique for measuring preferences in demographic studies. *Demography,* 1977, 14, 97-102.

Gagnon, J. H., and Simon, W. *Sexual conduct: The social sources of human sexuality.* Chicago: Aldine, 1973

Gecas, V. The influence of social class on socialization. In W. R. Burr, R. Hill, F. I. Nye, and I. L. Reiss (Eds.), *Contemporary theories about the family* (Vol. 1). New York: Free Press, 1979.

Gustavus, S. The family size preferences of young people: A replication of longitudinal follow-up study. *Studies in Family Planning,* 1973, 4, 335-342.

Gustavus, S. Fertility socialization research in the United States: A progress report. *Papers of the East-West Population Institute,* July 1975, 35.

Gustavus, S. O., and Nam, C. B. The formation and stability of ideal family size among young people. *Demography,* 1970, 7, 43-51.

Hobbs, D. F., Jr., and Cole, S. P. Transition to parenthood: A decade replication. *Journal of Marriage and the Family,* 1976, 38 723-731.

Hock, E., Christman, K., and Hock, M. Career-related decisions of mothers and infants. *Family Relations. Journal of Applied Family and Child Studies,* 1980, 29(3), 325-330.

Houseknecht, S. K. Timing of the decision to remain voluntarily childless: Evidence for continuous socialization. *Psychology of Women Quarterly,* 1979, 4, 81-96.

Houseknecht, S. K. Voluntary childlessness. In M. S. Sussman and S. K. Steimetz, *Handbook on marriage and the family.* Chicago: Rand McNally, forthcoming.

Johnson, N. E., and Stokes, C. S. Family size in successive generations: The effects of birth order, intergenerational change in lifestyle, and familial satisfaction. *Demography,* 1976, 13(2), 175-187.

Kidwell, J. S. Sibling size, spacing, sex and birth order: Their effects on perceived parent-adolescent relationships. *Journal of Marriage and the Family,* 1981, 43, forthcoming.

Lamb, M. E. The father's role in the infant's social world. In J. H. Stevens and M. Mathews (Eds.), *Mother/child, father/child relationships.* Washington, DC: National Association for the Education of Young Children, 1978.

LaRossa, R. *Conflict and power in marriage: Expecting the first child.* Beverly Hills, CA: Sage Publications, 1977

LeMasters, E. E. *Parents in modern America.* Homewood, IL: Dorsey, 1974.

McAllister, P., Stokes, C. S., and Knapp, M. Size of family of orientation, birth order, and fertility values: A re-examination. *Journal of Marriage and the Family,* 1974, 36, 337-342.

McGhee, P. E., and Frueh, T. Television viewing and the learning of sex-role stereotypes. *Sex Roles,* 1980, 6, 179-188.

Miller, B. C., and Sollie, D. L. Normal stresses during the transitions to parenthood. *Family Relations. Journal of Applied Family and Child Studies,* 1980, 29(4), 459-465.

Moore, K. A. *Policy determinants of adolescent pregnancy and childbearing.* Paper presented at the Contractor/Grantee Workshop on Adolescent Fertility Behavior, Center for Population Research of the National Institute for Child Health and Human Development, Bethesda, Maryland, 1980.

Otto, L. B. Antecendents and consequences of marital timing. In W. R Burr, R. Hill, F. I. Nye, and I. L. Reiss (Eds), *Contemporary theories about the family* (Vol. 1), New York: Free Press, 1979.

Philliber, S. G. A conceptual framework for population socialization. *Population and Environment,* 1980, 3(1), 3-9. (a)

Philliber, S. G. Socialization for childbearing. *Journal of Social Issues,* 1980, 36(1), 30-44. (b)

Presser, H. B. *Sex-role socialization for motherhood.* Paper presented at the annual meeting of the Population Association of America, New York, New York, 1974.

Presser, H. B. Social factors affecting the timing of the first child. In W. B. Miller and L. F. Newman (Eds.), *The first child and family formation,* Chapel Hill NC: Carolina Population Center, 1978.

Russell, C. S. Transition to parenthood: Problems and gratification. *Journal of Marriage and the Family,* 1974, 36, 294-302.

Russo, N. F., and Brackbill, Y. Population and youth. In J. T Fawcett (Ed.), *Psychological perspectives on population.* New York: Basic Books, 1973.

Scanzoni, J. *Sex roles, life styles, and childbearing: Changing patterns in marriage and the family.* New York: Free Press, 1975

Scanzoni, J., and Fox, G. L. Sex roles, family and society: The seventies and beyond. *Journal of Marriage and the Family,* 1980, 42, 743-756

Schvaneveldt, J. D., and Ihinger, M. Sibling relationships in the family. In W. R. Burr, R. Hill, F. I. Nye, and I. L. Reiss (Eds.), *Contemporary theories about the family* (Vol. 1). New York: Free Press, 1979.

Simmons, A. B., and Turner, J. E. The socialization of sex-roles and fertility ideals: A study of two generations in Toronto. *Journal of Comparative Family Studies,* 1976, 7(2), 255-271.

Spanier, G. B. Formal and informal sex education as determinants of premarital sexual behavior. *Archives of Sexual Behavior,* 1976, 5, 39-67.

Spanier, G. B. Sources of sex information and premarital sexual behavior. *Journal of Sex Research,* 1977, 13, 73-88.

Thornton, A. The influence of first generation fertility and economic status on second generation fertility. *Population and Environment,* 1980, 3(1), 51-72.

Troll, L., and Bengtson, V. Generations in the family. In W. R. Burr, R. Hill, F. I. Nye, and I. L. Reiss (Eds.), *Contemporary theories about the family* (Vol. 1). New York: Free Press, 1979.

Veevers, J. E. Voluntarily childless wives: An exploratory study. *Sociology and Social Research,* 1973, 57, 356-366.

Weiss, E., Kline, F. G., Rogers, E. M., Cohen, M. E., and Dodge, J. A. Communication and population socialization among youth: Communication Behavior and Family Planning Information. Paper presented at the annual meeting of the Population Association of America, New York, 1974.

Weitzman, L. J. *Sex role socialization.* Palo Alto, CA: Mayfield Publishing, 1979.

2

Sexual Decision-Making

ITS DEVELOPMENT AND DYNAMICS

Deborah I. Frank and John Scanzoni

Sexuality has always had a prominent place in religion, public morality, and law. If there was any realm where variability and discretion were formally prohibited and, hence, the need for decision-making was seemingly unnecessary, it was sexuality. In the Judeo-Christian tradition of Western society, strict norms prescribed chastity for the unmarried, fidelity for the married. One might assume that the moral norms were enough to compel comformity, but because of the great pleasure of sex, they were not. Therefore, added to the norms were strong legal and community sanctions against violators. The recent declines in the severity of those sanctions make more salient than ever before the significance of decision-making regarding potential sexual partners and decisions pertaining to specific behaviors know as "sexual gratifications."

Collins's (1975: 225) analysis makes it clear that prior to the modern era, virtually all aspects of women's lives — including sexual — were under the control of men. Men controlled "the scheduling of sexual intercourse and who gets most of the orgasms." Hence, both in terms of options regarding potential partners and in terms of dynamics of sexual satisfactions, the processes of sexual decision-making were significantly affected by women's disadvantaged position. A third area of women's disadvantage is pregnancy risk, as illustrated by Byrne's (1979: 305) observation that "most people are found not to use any form of contraception when they first engage in sexual intercourse. . . . There are no role models and no imaginative cues to suggest the inclusion of contraception as a part of sexuality."

Because many women in modern society have access to economic resources, they "become at least potentially free to negotiate [these three aspects of] their own sexual relationships" (Collins, 1975: 243). Although most women do not yet earn as much money as the men with whom they interact, Collins (1975: 250) points out the decisions are being made based on "income resources as well as sexual attractiveness, social status, personal compatibility, deference and emotional support. The greater freedom of women from economic dependence on men means that: sexual bargaining can be less concerned with marriage; dating can go on as a form of short-run bargaining, in which both [sexes] trade on their own attractiveness or capacity to entertain in return for sexual favors and/or being entertained. Where women bring economic resources of their own, they may concentrate on bargaining for sexual attractiveness on the part of men."

In short, it seems apparent that the sexual situation among contemporary young adults is moving away from regulations and prescriptions based on traditional norms. What is emerging instead are much more fluid arrangements based on the dynamics of the partners' decision-making. However, those dynamics have never been thoroughly analyzed and dissected. The purpose of this chapter is to analyze those dynamics, with particular focus on three issues: partner selection, gratification, and contraception among young adults.

Applying Gulliver (1979), furthermore, we analyze sexual decision-making in terms of both its developmental and its cyclical components. The developmental refers to the stages of the partners' relationship and might be compared to the scenes of a live play. On the other hand, the cyclical, or what Blalock and Wilken (1979) call the reciprocal, refers to the specific interactions between the partners and might be compared to the dialogue and other behaviors and communications between actors within each scene of a play.

DEVELOPMENTAL STAGES

The developmental scenes or stages of any relationship have been described as exploration, expansion, and commitment — or an evolution from low to high mutual interdependence (Scanzoni, 1979). Analogously, Money (1976, 1980) identifies three levels of increasing "pair bonding" within the sexual relationship — proceptive, acceptive, and conceptive. The two developmental sequences can be related as follows: First, the exploration stage of any relationship subsumes attraction and learning about the other to see if the relationship might be pursued (Scanzoni, 1979). Similarly, the proceptive stage of the sexual relationship is the erotic process of attraction, during which the couple engages in certain "courtship" behaviors and ponders whether or not they will have a sexual relationship (Money, 1976: 274).

Second, the acceptive stage is the culmination of the proceptive phase in that coitus takes place. Having accepted each other, the couple is sharing the responsiblity of giving each other maximal erotic experience. Acceptive activity may very well be the catalyst that facilitates development of the couple's overall relationship from the exploration to the expansion stage. The latter stage is marked by increasing investments in the relationship, resulting in greater interdependence of mutual interests and goals (Scanzoni, 1979: 79).

Third, the commitment stage, according to Scanzoni, represents the greatest level of interdependence within the overall relationship and is characterized by a high level of mutual inputs, consistently invested over time. High interdependence also characterizes third sexual or conceptive stage, which emerges with conception or pregnancy and the potential of parenthood (Money, 1976: 276). If we combine Money's three sexual stages with Scanzoni's three general relationship stages, we arrive at three categories describing the ongoing development (or scenes) of a sexual relationship: proceptive/exploration, acceptive/expansion, and conceptive/commitment.

RECIPROCAL DYNAMICS

Besides sequential stages, the remaining aspect of decision-making is what occurs *between* partners *within* each stage or scene. Analogous to an actual play, these dynamics contribute to the progression (or lack of it) from one stage to the next. Before we examine how the reciprocal dynamics influence the evolution between the three stages or categories, we must briefly examine the nature of the dynamics themselves.

Figure 2.1 shows that reciprocal dynamics can be subdivided into three components: context, processes, and outcomes (Scanzoni and Szinovacz, 1980). The first component is the social setting, or *context*,

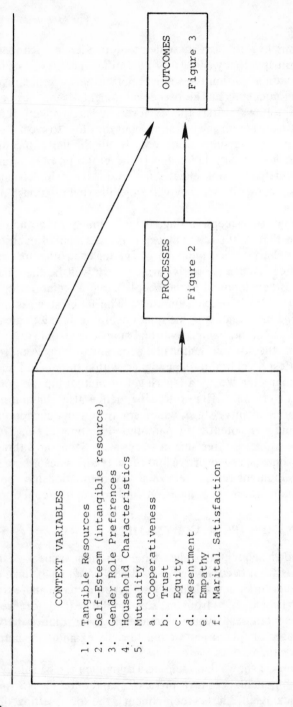

Figure 2.1 Elements of an Explicit Decision-Making Model
SOURCE: Adapted from Scanzoni and Szinovacz, 1980.

which comprises the variables displayed in Figure 2.1, including the degree of mutuality. Mutuality consists of variables (such as trust, cooperativeness, and resentment) emerging from past decision-making processes and subsequently influencing current decision-making processes, thus forging a significant link between past and present decision-making.

The second component in Figure 2.1 — *explicit processes* — is elaborated in Figure 2.0. It is by tracing the processes of who said what and how it was said that the cyclical or reciprocal nature of (sexual) decision-making can be most sharply observed. Figure 2.2 illustrates the sequential nature of these interactions. For example, Actor (A) may initiate a request to Other (O) regarding a certain sexual matter subsumed under partners, gratifications, or contraception. If O reciprocates with a "yes," the matter has been "decided" and is presumably "settled"; hence, that brief cycle is over. However, O might respond with a "yes, but" or a "no," followed by his/her own sequential messages, which would also follow the reciprocal dynamics indicated in Figure 2.2.

As noted in Figure 2.2, point 5, based on the sorts of responses A and O give each other, we can grasp their interaction processes in four ways. One is *compliance*, or a "yes." A second is *discussion*, or a series of "yes, but's." Third is *conflict and negotiation*, or a series of "no" responses. Also, there may be "mixed" discussion and conflict.

Finally, as Figure 2.1 shows, the context and processes give rise to variation in the partners' perceived decision-making *outcomes*, which is displayed in Figure 2.3.

Implicit Processes. Strauss (1978) argues that some persons communicate and organize their relationships apart from the kinds of verbal cycles just described. The dimension of implicitness that is most easily grasped is that of *spontaneous consensus*, in which, as a result of shared preferences, parties concur on a set of actions, even though they have never verbalized them. A *tacit understanding* occurs when each becomes aware that the other prefers an alternative; however, they do not discuss or negotiate it. On the one hand, they may have never discussed it, yet their tacitness emerges through unspoken cues and clues. On the other hand, at some prior distant time, they may have been explicit about a matter whose out come either remained in flux or was regulated (Figure 2.3); but because they have been silent for a long time, the matter may be said to have developed into a tacit understanding. Human sexuality issues can

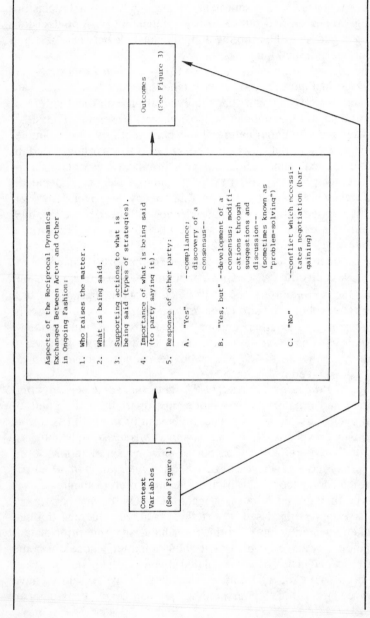

Aspects of the Reciprocal Dynamics
Exchanged Between Actor and Other
in Ongoing Fashion:

1. Who raises the matter.

2. What is being said.

3. Supporting actions to what is
   being said (types of strategies).

4. Importance of what is being said
   (to party saying it).

5. Response of other party:

   A. "Yes"   --compliance;
                   discovery of a
                   consensus--

   B. "Yes, but" --development of a
                   consensus; modifi-
                   cations through
                   suggestions and
                   discussion--
                   (sometimes known as
                   "problem-solving")

   C. "No"   --conflict which necessi-
                   tates negotiation (bar-
                   gaining)

Context
Variables

(See Figure 1)

Outcomes

(See Figure 3)

Figure 2.2 Component Variables Located in the Social Processes Segment of the Decision-Making Model
SOURCE: Adapted from Scanzoni and Szinovacz, 1980.

A. CONSENSUS

Agreements Preceded by Either Discussion or Negotiation or Both.

B. UNITS IN FLUX

1. Discussions or Negotiations are Continuing
2. Agree to Disagree

C. CONFLICT-REGULATION

1. One party continues attempts to negotiate; the other does not.
2. One party effectively prohibits the other party from continuing negotiations.

RESOLUTION — Effective Decision-Making

REGULATION — Ineffective Decision-Making

Figure 2.3   A Continuum of Decision-Making Outcomes
SOURCE: Adapted from Scanzoni and Szinovacz, 1980.

evolve in either direction — from explicit to implicit or from implicit to explicit.

APPLYING THE MODEL

Proceptive Exploratory Stage

Having briefly described the basic elements of the decision-making model, We shall illustrate it by simultaneously considering both the sequential stages and the reciprocal dynamics, with special concern for how the latter influences the former.

When a couple initially meet, factors such as physical attractiveness, surface behaviors, and similar interests lead each person to weigh the potential rewards and costs of a mutual relationship in comparison to those of current relationships (Adams, 1979). The exploratory phase of a relationship is a time to validate these initial impressions and decide whether to continue the relationship by making investments into it (Scanzoni, 1979). According to Money (1980), proception includes direct or subtle verbal and nonverbal cues. Flirting, eye contact, tone of voice, or pressure of a touch may communicate sexual interest and receptivity, as might more obvious behaviors of necking, petting, and foreplay. This proceptive stage may last a very short time, a few hours, or longer, perhaps years. Its ending is marked by having or not having coitus. Sexual decision-making during the proceptive stage is unique in that the pair has no previous mutual sexual history. Thus, each individual's resources, sex role preferences, and prior sexual experiences, along with the attributions attached to Other's behaviors and intentions, weigh heavily on the attraction process itself.

Explicit and Compliant Processes

When an explicit coital request is made and Other says yes, it is likely that both partners possess comparable levels of tangible and intangible resources, such as self-esteem (Scanzoni and Szinovacz, 1980). If those levels are high, each is likely to feel that she/he can form alternative relationships that are potentially just as rewarding. Thus, A verbalizes his/her request for coitus, perceiving that it will have rewards and negligible costs for him/her, while O accepts, anticipating similar satisfactions, and knowing that if she/he did not accept, the costs involved would still be minimal.

Similarity in sex role preferences and related sexual values should also increase mutual attraction (Scanzoni and Szinovacz, 1980; Adams, 1979) and influence the likelihood of having coitus. For example, the woman who holds egalitarian sex role preferences, and who believes that coitus should be as pleasurable for her as for him, is likely to comply with his initiative primarily because she feels it will be enjoyable for her, not out of traditional female concerns that sex is *the* way to "get a man." Murstein and Holden (1979) found that premarital sexual activity is associated with liberal philosophies about sex: Sex for "fun" is "OK" if it is part of a "good" relationship. Regen (1978) concludes that attraction will be increased if A believes that O's positive actions are directed uniquely toward him/her and are based on an accurate assessment of his/her characteristics. Thus, if both engage in conversation and interaction that indicate their attention to each other as valued, unique persons, and that also promote the perceptions of commonalities, it appears the likelihood of eventual agreement to have coitus is increased. In effect, these interactions allow each person to make attributions regarding whether Other would be a potentially desirable mate in a rewarding relationship. Prior sexual decisioning will also play a major role in forming attributions regarding the desirability of Other as potential sexual partner. For example, previous positive sexual experiences are likely to increase current receptivity to coitus when there are many similarities between the past and current interaction. If the current interaction is perceived to be very different from past negative experiences, this too could increase willingness to comply.

Implicit and Compliant Processes

In addition to the dynamics just described, the decision to have sexual intercourse can be the result of *spontaneous consensus*. This occurs when the parties share similar perceptions regarding the role of coitus within a relationship — when it should occur, under what circumstances, and what it means. A certain amount of interaction (verbal and nonverbal) takes place during the parties' initial meeting, during which each may attribute to the other norms and preferences similar to his/her own. If there is similarity it becomes likely that when the purely nonverbal proceptive-type behaviors are initiated, they will be reciprocated and culminate in coitus. Results from a survey of *Cosmopolitan'* readers (an admittedly biased sample of

21-35-year-old, well-educated, mostly single women) illustrate this sort of spontaneous consensus. According to Wolfe's (1980: 264-265) analysis, the respondents "view sex as a pleasure in and of itself, a way of enriching their lives . . . and 97% enjoy making love always or at least usually." Further, "men have become so accustomed to a woman who says 'yes' with no thought other than going to bed, that they assume every woman is like that. You can't say no without their thinking you're weird or a prude. So you do it." Thus, it would seem that these women and the men they date hold expectations that sex *will occur* and *not be refused* and also *will be enjoyable* for both. The decision has been made implicitly and the proceptive-type behaviors serve only as precursors to the often inevitable outcome of coitus.

The prior quotations suggest there are times when the woman (or man), though complying, is nonetheless aware that she (he) would rather refuse. In those instances, actual preferences are kept silent, owing to perceived costs, such as embarrassment, peer ostracism, feeling deviant, or fearing partner's rejection and loss of the entire relationship while having no alternatives to it. Justifications for the silence and compliance are attributed to the uniqueness of the situation ("it just happened" or "I wouldn't have but I had too much to drink"), to social norms ("everyone else does, so I might as well too"), or to unique traits of the partner that make the compliance a special situation ("I usually don't have sex the first night, but he was so nice and I felt so close to him it seemed natural to go ahead").

Compliance Processes and Contraception

When there is compliance to the coital request, a contraceptive decision occurs simultaneously either explicitly or implicitly. When the explicit sexual request receives an immediate yes, the contraceptive decision may spring from spontaneous consensus. For example, if the pair are alike in resources, sex role preferences, and the extent of their prior sexual activity, they may attribute similar expectations to each other. Perhaps the man implicitly assumes she is on the Pill and otherwise would not have said "yes," so he does not explicitly concern himself with the contraceptive issue (Luker, 1975). Based on her prior sexual experiences (which have taught her that men expect sexually active women to be on the Pill), the woman has become a regular Pill user. The pair never verbalize the decision to use contraceptives. Rather, it is made via spontaneous consensus in that both "know" the woman will take the necessary measures.

As with coitus itself, persons may keep their *actual* contraceptive preferences silent. For instance, the woman might prefer to use a particular device she has or to suggest her mate us a certain method, or she may want to delay coitus until she does obtain the "right" contraceptive. However, she may not verbalize any of these preferences if she perceives that he might be displeased with "a break in the action" or "destroying the mood" (Gemme, 1980). Failure to verbalize preferences is also likely if the woman perceives rejection owing to her suggestion that the man take part in providing protection or that they delay intercourse. Furthermore, if the woman does not define herself as sexually active, making contraceptive matters explicit may result in dissonance between her own self-image and the one implied by that sort of explicit discussion. Finally, it may be that getting pregnant is not perceived as costly if she views abortion as a acceptable option. The woman might even be indifferent to the costs of pregnancy, should that occur. Any or all of these contingencies may lead some women to perceive no reason to risk losing immediate and possible long-term rewards by making their contraceptive preferences explicit.

Discussion and/or Conflict Processes

If O responds "yes, but" or "no" to A's sexual invitation or contraceptive plans, O is likely to have comparable resources enabling O to risk the costs of potential displeasure or rejection. The outcome (Figure 2.3) of those negotiation processes can be a resolution of the issue (for example, to have coitus and use condoms); to agree to disagree on contraception but to go ahead and have coitus; or some form of conflict regulation in which O or A unilaterally imposes his/her will regarding coitus and/or contraception. Take, for example, the woman on a college scholarship who is not using contraceptives, yet is against abortion. She begins engaging in non verbal proceptive behaviors with her boyfriend, who subsequently indicates, also implicitly, his desire for intercourse. The decisioning cycle continues as she responds non verbally by trying to manage his sexual advances — implicitly indicating she does not want coitus. If this is not effective, the strength of her educational aspirations and her antiabortion preferences motivate her to become explicit and verbalize "I can't — I don't want to get pregnant." Or she might respond with a "yes, but" and delay having coitus until she obtains the Pill. He might concur with her, or he might ignore her verbal inputs and attempt to regulate (dominate) their conflict by coercing her into coitus by threatening to leave the relationship. Or he may escalate the conflict by using physical coercion to achieve coitus without her actual consent. Seventy-five percent of *Cosmopolitan* readers report they have been bullied into making love, while a quarter report rape. Of the latter, 51 percent were raped by friends (Wolfe, 1980).

Assuming physical coercion does not occur, A's perception that she/he has resources to pursue alternative relationships affects continued negotiation regarding coitus. The importance attributed to sex may determine whether or not the relationship ends or whether a *tacit understanding* evolves where both know, but do not discuss, the fact that one wants coitus and the other does not (or does not until specified conditions are met). Nevertheless, because the understanding is maintained apart from coitus, and thus other types of rewards are exchanged, the relationship may gradually evolve into the expansion or even commitment stages. By this means it is quite possible for the overall relationship to develop beyond its exploratory phase, even though sexually the couple may not have completed the proceptive stage. Conversely, a couple may experience coitus and thus complete the proceptive stage, but their overall relationship may never evolve into the expansion phase.

Acceptive Expansion Stage

The expansion phase of relationship development in Scanzoni's formulation is characterized by the emergence of mutual goals, a sense of trust, and maximum joint profit. In Money's formulation, couples enter the acceptive stage of their sexual relationship following their initial coitus, and their acceptive experiences may, or may not, enhance the expansion of their overall relationship. Since the prime focus of the acceptive stage is the fostering of maximum erotic experience for each partner (Money, 1976: 274), it follows that the greater the sexual enjoyments they experience, the greater the likelihood of expansion throughout their overall relationship. Not only does the acceptive phase differ from the proceptive in *focus,* it also differs because now couples possess a shared history on which to base their current decision-making. But like the proceptive stage, the acceptive must be understood in terms of a *developmental* notion. That is, if the particular decisioning reciprocities are effective and the couple's sexual experiences are satisfactory, then their relationship is likely eventually to evolve into one based on commitment. Conversely, ineffectiveness and dissatisfaction could result in the relationship's termination.

Explicit Processes and
Sexual Satisfaction

Walen (1980) defines a positive sexual experience as one with a playful, relaxed attitude and minimal emotional distress. However, often the pair's first sexual experience is not totally pleasurable because of the anxiety associated with an unfamiliar sex partner (Masters and Johnson, 1970). Thus, one or both partners may desire explicit discussions regarding how to foster mutual pleasure during subsequent sexual activity. This is especially pertinent in view of the prevailing norm in Western society that sexual interaction should provide orgasm/ejaculation and be a *totally* pleasurable experience. Hence A may ask O what his/her preferences are, or ask for validation that what she/he has done is enjoyable. During those communications, if both persons have a positive self-concept they are each likely to make and also to comply with explicit requests pertaining to their sexual activity. For example, the woman who possesses the resource of knowledge regarding her own sexual responses is more likely to indicate her preference for a certain kind of stimulation (Barbach, 1976); the more positive the man's self-concept, the less likely he is to feel threatened by her request and thus the more likely he is to comply with it. Hence, the woman becomes more likely to reciprocate in kind. Agreement on sex role preferences has a profound impact on acceptive-stage decisioning. For instance, the egalitarian female who rejects the double standard is more likely to make explicit requests for sexual satisfactions (Barbach, 1980), and the nontraditional male is more likely to comply. While this open kind of sexual communication may not yet be the actual behavior for the majority of couples, increasingly more persons are espousing the value of this explicitness.

Explicit Processes and
Contraception

Either the failure to resolve the contraceptive issue satisfactorily during proception, or a desire to renegotiate it, may prompt one or both partners to pursue it during the acceptive phase. For example, if a couple has ignored contraception during proception, the newly increased risk of pregnancy owing to more frequent intercourse may influence a woman with resources comparable to those of her partner to raise or renegotiate the issue of effective contraception. If contraception did occur during proception it was likely through the male's use of condoms or withdrawal (Fox, 1974). But as the couple's sexual relationship becomes more regularized and increased erotic pleasure becomes a more central goal of this developmental stage, it becomes likely that the man (or the woman) will make the suggestion that she become primarily responsible for contraception through the use of means that are coitus-independent (Chilman, 1978; Cvetkovich and Grote, 1977). Since maximum sexual pleasure and effective contraception are so closely interwoven, it follows that the same sorts of context variables that promote decision-making resulting in optimal pleasure will promote decision-making resulting in effective contraception as well.

Implicit Understandings

While a certain proportion of couples achieve mutually satisfactory agreements regarding sexual satisfactions and contraception as they move through the acceptive/expansion stage, many others do not. One reason they do not is the failure to verbalize preferences even though their sexual experiences have become regularized. As in the proceptive stage, disparity of resources (tangible and intangible) is one major factor preventing explicit communication of sexual preferences. The partner sensing power asymmetry in their overall relationship (most often the woman; Collins, 1975) is more likely to comply (with male sexual preferences) than she/he is to make requests of her/his own (Barbach, 1976).

Furthermore, Masters and Johnson (1970) argue that fear of rejection inhibits expressing sexual preferences. Even some avant garde *Cosmopolitan* women with obvious resources expressed shyness about indicating their sexual preferences lest they "injure" the male ego and alienate their partners (Wolfe, 1980). Moreover, the more traditional A's and O's sex-role preferences, the less likely it is that the woman's sexual wishes will be freely expressed (Rubin, 1976). For example, gender-traditional couples are more likely to have a tacit understanding that the male is well-versed in the art of sexual pleasuring. For the woman to tell him or actually show him during coitus what she likes might tend to destroy the image that each has of his sexual prowess (Zilbergeld, 1978). Moreover, the female who perceives that her man wants a "good" woman (not "sexually experienced") may not indicate her sexual preferences, lest he think less of her because of her sexual awareness (Lobitz and Lobitz, 1978). Finally, if the overall expanding relationship is a rewarding one, A can justify his/her silence in sexual matters by reasoning that O's inputs are acceptable — better than previous relationships and perhaps better than possible alternatives. Hence, why risk the jeopardizing nonsexual benefits of the overall relationship?

Similar reasoning appears to explain failure to express contraceptive preferences, even during the acceptive phase. Furthermore, in a relationship that is merely midway (expansion) in its overall development, the risks of explicitly disagreeing about contraception might be perceived as greater than the risks of getting pregnant. For example, Wolfe (1980) noted that 38 percent of her female respondents not using contraceptives were between the ages of 30 and 34, and she suggests they might be trying to get pregnant. Perhaps because of their age, these women may perceive conception as unlikely, abortion as a viable alternative to an unwanted conception, or conception as a possible means to secure a committed relationship (50 percent of Wolfe's respondents expressed disillusionment with the lack of emotional involvement they felt with their mates).

Discussion/Conflict
Processes

A high degree of perceived anxiety, inequity, and sexual dissatisfaction (in conjunction with comparable resources and egalitarian sex-role preferences) are likely to stimulate explicit discussions and often disagreements regarding sexual satisfactions and contraception. The cyclical content of these decisioning processes depends on the attributions A makes concerning *why* O raised the issue and *how* its resolution might subsequently affect the relationship. Harvey et al. (1978) report that women and men diverge significantly in their sexual satisfaction levels. Moreover, they also differ in how important sexual issues are compared to other issues in their overall relationship.

Orvis et al. (1976) report that among certain cohabiting and "steadily dating" couples, partners tend to differ over the meaning of conflict: A tends to see it as a means to resolve a particular issue, but O sees it as rejection of his/her and their total relationship. Consequently, disagreements are most likely to be made explicit when the relationship is well into the acceptive phase and one or both perceive it to be in their best interests to clarify and understand O's behavior (Orvis et al., 1976). If the male is told he is not being affectionate enough, he may try to resist that "designation" (Prus, 1979) via several strategies. On the other hand, he might accept the designation and suggest a compromise. The outcome of this explicit decisioning is then shaped through their context factors — including their mutuality. Rusbaut (1980) suggests that willingness to remain in a relationship during its acceptive/expansion phases is motivated by the number of investments one has made in it, as well as the reward/cost balance and available alternatives. Accordingly, if investments in the relationship are perceived as minimal, then termination might occur in the wake of regulated sexual conflicts (high costs), expecially if an attractive alternative is readily apparent.

Conceptive/Commitment Stage

If ongoing reciprocities become sufficiently great, the overall relationship gradually evolves into what was defined earlier as the *commitment* stage. In the literature, the notion of commitment is often pictured in static terms, as a pinnacle toward which partners strive. Once there, a couple's level of commitment seemingly ceases to fluctuate or, if it shifts, to move only toward a lower degree of commitment. But such a static conception is hardly relevant to contemporary sexual and marital patterns, especially in light of the two related issues analyzed in this segment: marital sexual satisfaction and extramarital coitus (Swidler, 1980). Similarly, what Money (1976, 1980) labels the *conceptive* phase must also be thought of in dynamic, not static, terms. For example, newly married couples (presumably located within the commitment stage) face "conceptive" questions concerning how many, if any, children to have; when to have them; how to care for the child if both parents work; and what contraceptives to use prior to when they begin trying to conceive.

The couple carries into the conceptive/commitment stage a relatively extensive decisioning history, especially if their marriage was preceded by sexual activity or by cohabitation. Mutuality levels are relatively high, or presumably they would not have formalized their commitment.[1] Assuming they have never explicitly discussed the possibility of being child-free (Polonko, 1979), each may assume they will one day have children. However, the woman may wish to delay the first child indefinitely, while the man may prefer to have one as soon as possible. The catalyst for making that implicit divergence explicit is, of course, contraception. He verbalizes the suggestion that they stop (or not start) using contraceptives, in order to conceive. If her sex role preferences are less traditional than his, and she wishes to pursue educational or occupational opportunities instead of immediate motherhood, regulated conflict in this situation is a likely possibility. The negative impact of this regulated conflict on sexual satisfaction may be twofold: First, lack of resolution over any matter can create resentment that undermines desire to give maximum erotic satisfaction to one's partner. Second, since the conflict is over a matter intrinsic to coitus, the unwillingness to provide erotic pleasure may be intensified.

The preceding processes may occur prior to the first child, and very early in marriage. However, recent government data showing an increase in childbearing among women in their late twenties and early thirties suggest that similar processes could erupt prior to a first birth much later in the marriage. The matter may be regulated by one partner early in marriage and maintained for several years therafter. A variation on the conflict could apply to the issue of an additional child at that same later marital stage. Complicating any conceptive decision at that later point is the gradual winding down of the biological time clock. In another vein, some couples experience unintended pregnancies (Westoff and Ryder, 1977), and the discovery of conception by a couple where A does not want the child and prefers abortion could result in regulated conflict if O resists abortion and instead wants a child. In yet another situation, Kolodny et al. (1979) suggest that couples who have delayed pregnancy for some years, and then begin to try (unsuccessfully) to conceive may experience a decline in their sexual satisfaction. The reason, they say, is the couple's emphasis on "getting down to business" and their tendency to make pleasuring secondary. The chief aim of coitus becomes conception, rather than erotic satisfaction.

According to Westoff and Ryder (1977) voluntary sterilization (vasectomy or tubal ligation) has become the most frequently used method of contraception among persons over age 30. The decision to become sterile means, of course, the termination of the conceptive stage. However, the effects of that termination on a couple's commitment to their relationship can either be positive or negative, depending on their mutuality, as well as on similarities and differences in other context variables, such as tangible and intangible resources and sex role preferences. In the same vein, the effect is more likely to be positive if the sterilization decision itself was characterized by a consensus rather than a conflict-regulation outcome.

In contrast, couples who remain fecund past the attainment of their desired family size continue to face the possibility of contraception emerging as a conflict issue (relating to type of method, including sterilization and abortion, the Pill's side effects, and so forth), which in turn could undermine sexual satisfaction. In any case, once the conceptive phase is completed (non fecund), or is in "remission" (fecund), couples may face many years throughout which sexual satisfaction continues as a live decisioning issue along with, according to several analysts (Reiss, 1980; Libby and Whitehurst, 1979), the related and increasingly salient option of extramarital coitus.

During this potentially lengthy period, certain couples may feel that sexual experimentation within marriage or with extramarital coitus is simply irrelevant. Sexual decisioning is based on their implicit consensus that "sex has always been good this way, so why change?" In contrast, couples who are explicit regarding their sexual preferences report a greater degree of sexual satisfaction (Sarrel and Sarrel, 1980; Heath, 1978). The fact that increasing numbers of women are entering the labor force while still in the conceptive phase may contribute to a heightened explicitness. Greater tangible resources along with enhanced self-esteem (as a result of job performance and potential alternative relationships) may encourage the woman to be assertive in requesting greater erotic inputs from her spouse. Sarrell and Sarrell (1980) suggest that the kinds of inputs most frequently discussed are increased coital frequency and oral-genital stimulation. Heath (1978) concludes that the more couples have over the years increased their mutuality (especially trust), the more likely they are to risk (temporarily) "hurting" their partners by making the sexual preferences explicit. But there is a sharp contrast between the legitimacy of expressing preferences for increased erotic pleasure from one's spouse and verbally expressing preferences for extramarital coitus. Sarrel and Sarrel (1980) report that only 16 percent of their respondents are afraid to risk rejection by requesting greater sexual satisfactions from their spouse, while Reiss (1980) reports that fewer than 10 percent of couples explicitly negotiate extramarital coitus. Furthermore, several opinion surveys report that Americans overwhelmingly disapprove of extramarital coitus (Wolfe, 1980; Reiss, 1980; Wachowiak and Bragg, 1980). Nevertheless, the earlier Kinsey et al. (1948) data and the current Wolfe (1980) report (69 percent of the working women in the latter study had extramarital coitus) suggest that a certain proportion of married persons are deciding unilaterally to engage in extramarital behavior without, apparently, making that explicit to their spouses.

Both sexual satisfaction and extramarital coitus are linked to the ongoing development of the couple's larger commitment to each other. The assumption made most often in the literature (Walster et al., 1978; Smith and Smith, 1974) is that declines in sexual (along with other marital) satisfactions signal decreasing commitment to the overall relationship. This decreased commitment influences A to take the risks inherent in extramarital coitus, but not to take added risks intrinsic to making the issue part of explicit decision-making with his/her spouse. A second pattern (Reiss, 1980) is also presumably associated with declining commitment. O knows that A is having extramarital coitus, but in spite of O's ongoing explicit negotiations to get A to stop, A persists, and thus regulated conflict is the result. A third pattern is a variant of the second in that after a period of time, O may cease to make the matter a verbal issue and instead simply tacitly concur with it — there is toleration but silent disapproval. Of course in some cases there may be tacit acceptance quite apart from prior verbal negotiation.

Judge Ben Lindsey observed in 1927 "that such tacit agreements are far more common than even students of these matters have any idea of" (Smith and Smith, 1974: Ch. 5). Certainly far less common is what Smith and Smith (1974: 21) call "transmarital sexuality." Here the couple have explicitly negotiated and agreed that one (but usually both) can engage in sex with someone other than the spouse. Often (but not necessarily) A's sexual activity takes place with O present, such as at a "swinging" party. But whether the partner is present or not, the assumption underlying this fourth situation, in contrast to the other three, is that there has been no necessary decline in commitment to the overall marital relationship (Libby and Whitehurst, 1979). The argument is that since they arrived at a joint decision regarding the matter, their total commitment is presumably enhanced, as would be the case when any matter of extreme gravity is effectively negotiated. Less considered, however, is the developmental nature of such an agreement. Some months or years after the agreement, A may wish to renegotiate the extramarital behavior and remove it from his/her relationship with O. If O resists, the consequences of that sort of necessarily highly emotionally charged conflict could have particularly negative consequences for the couple's reciprocal sexual inputs, as well as their overall marital commitment.

If sexual as well as other kinds of marital satisfactions gradually deteriorate (for whatever reason) during this state, the couple's commitment may eventually decline sufficiently to lead them to separation and/or divorce (Frank and Kupfer, 1976). Nevertheless, the evolution of one relationship to its extinction potentially sets in motion a new set of developmental processes, since one or both partners are likely to commence at the proceptive/exploratory stage with someone else (Glick and Norton, 1977). Conversely, rather than dissolve their relationship, a couple may simply tolerate an array of regulated sexual conflicts if other aspects of their relationship are satisfying. Finally, some couples may be able to carry on indefinitely the sorts of sexual decision-making that result in increased feeling of mutuality, interdependence, and sexual intimacy. Thus, their overall commitment is maintained and, in some instances, enhanced. Logically, those processes could occur in either monogamous or non-monogamous arrangements.

SUMMARY

Sexual decision-making was examined as a special case of social decision-making. Relationships were analyzed in terms of three major *developmental* categories. Evolution between categories takes place as a result of cyclical interaction processes occurring within categories between the partners. The particular issues examined were subsumed under choice of sexual partners, sexual satisfaction, and contraception. Clinical, sociological, and psychological literatures were used as bases for the decision-making model. The model can be applied in clinical settings as a basis for therapy, and in research settings as a source of testable hypotheses.

NOTE

1. As discussed in Scanzoni (1979), it is sometimes possible to enter legal marriage apart from commitment. For example, an adolescent woman, upon discovering she is pregnant, may be coerced into marriage because of parental pressures.

REFERENCES

Adams, B. Mate selection in the United States: A theoretical summarization. In W. R. Burr, R. Hill, F. I. Nye, and I. L. Reiss (Eds.), *Contemporary theories about the family* (Vol. 1). New York: Free Press, 1979, 259-265.

Barbach, L. *For yourself: The fulfillment of female sexuality.* New York: Anchor, 1976.

Barbach, L. *Women discover orgasm.* New York: Free Press, 1980.

Blalock, H. M., and Willkin, P. H. *Intergroup processes: A micro-macro perspective.* New York: Free Press, 1979.

Byrne, D. Determinants of contraceptive values and practices. In M. Cook and G. Wilson (Eds.), *Love and attraction.* New York: Pergamon, 1979.

Chilman, C. *Adolescent sexuality in a changing American Society: Social and psychological perspectives.* DHEW Publication (NIH) 79-1426.0, 1978, 3-154.

Collins, R. *Conflict sociology.* New York: Academic Press, 1975.

Cvetkovich, G., and Grote, B. *Adolescent development and teenage fertility.* Paper presented at the Planned Parenthood Regional Conference on Adolescence, Boise, Idaho, 1977.

Fox, G. L. Pragmatics, powerlessness and resentment: The female response to the male role in contraception. Paper presented at Groves Conference on Marriage and the Family, Hot Springs, Arkansas, 1974.

Frank, E., and Kupfer, D. In every marriage there are two marriages. *Journal of Sex and Marital Therapy,* 1976, 2 (Summer), 137-143.

Gemme, R. Some sexological aspects of contraception. *Journal of Sex Education and Therapy,* Summer, 1980 20-21.

Glick, P. C., and Norton, A. J. *Marrying, divorcing and living together in the U.S. today.* Washington, DC: Population Reference Bureau, 1977.

Gulliver, P. *Disputes and negotiations: A cross-cultural perspective.* New York: Academic Press, 1979.

Harvey, J., Wells, G., and Alvarez, M. Attribution in the context of conflict and separation in close relationships. In J. Harvey, W. Ickes, and R. Kidd (Eds.), *New directions in attribution research* (Vol. 2). New York: Wiley, 1978, 235-260.

Heath, D. Marital sexual enjoyment and frustration of professional men. *Archives of Sexual Behavior.* 1978, 7, 463-476.

Kinsey, A. C., Pomeroy, W. B., and Martin, C. E. *Sexual behavior in the human male.* Philadelphia: W. B. Saunders, 1948.

Kolodny, R., Masters, W., Johnson, V., and Biggs, M. Sex and family planning. *In Textbook of human sexuality for nurses.* Boston: Little, Brown, 1979, 279-322.

Libby, R. W., and Whitehurst, R. N. *Marriage and alternatives: Exploring intimate relationships.* Glenview, IL: Scott, Foresman, 1979.

Lobitz, C., and Lobitz, G. Clinical assessment in the treatment of sexual dysfunction. In J. LoPiccolo and L. LoPiccolo (Eds.), *Handbook of sex therapy.* New York: Plenum, 1978, 85-102.

Luker, K. *Taking chances: Abortion and the decision not to contracept.* Berkeley: University of California Press, 1975.

Masters, W., and Johnson, V. *Human sexual inadequacy,* Boston: Little, Brown, 1970.

Money, J. Sex, love and commitment. *Journal of Sex and Marital Therapy,* 1976, 2 (Winter), 273-276.

Money, J. *Love and love sickness: The science of sex, gender difference and pair bonding.* Baltimore: Johns Hopkins University Press, 1980, 73-104.

Murstein, B., and Holden, C. Sexual behavior and correlates among college students. *Adolescence,* 1979, 14, 625-639.

Orvis, B., Kelley, H., and Butler, D. Attributional conflict in young couples. In J. Harvey, W. Ickes, and R. Kidd (Eds.), *New directions in attribution research* (Vol. I). New York: Wiley, 1976, 353-386.

Polonko, K. *Accounting for the conditions of voluntary childlessness.* Unpublished doctoral dissertation, Indiana University, 1979.

Prus, R. Resisting designations: An extension of attribution theory into a negotiated context. *Sociologic Inquiry,* 1979, 45, 3-14.

Regen, D. Attributional aspects of interpersonal attraction. In J. Harvey, W Ickes, and R. Kidd (Eds.), *New directions in attribution research* (Vol. 2). New York: Wiley, 1978, 207-233.

Reiss, I. The sexual drives of married people: Inside and outside of marriage. In *Family Systems in America.* New York: Holt, Rinehart, & Winston, 1980, 271-315.

Rubin, L. B. *Worlds of pain: Life in the working-class.* New York: Basic Books, 1976.

Rusbaut, C. Commitment and satisfaction in romantic associations: A test of the investment model. *Journal of Experimental Social Psychology,* 1980, 16, 172-186.

Sarrel, P., and Sarrel, L. The *Redbook* report on sexual relationships. *Redbook,* October 1980, 72-80.

Scanzoni, J. Social exchange and behavioral interpendence. In T.L. Huston and R.L. Burgess (Eds.), *Social exchange and developing relationships.* New York: Academic Press, 1979, 61-98.

Scanzoni, J., and Szinovacz, M. *Family decision-making: A developmental sex-role model.* Beverly Hills, CA: Sage Publications, 1980.

Smith, J. R., and Smith, L. G. *Beyond monogamy: Recent studies of sexual alternatives in marriage.* Baltimore: Johns Hopkins University Press, 1974.

Strauss, A. *Negotiations: Varieties, contexts, processes and social order.* San Francisco: Jossey-Bass, 1978.

Swidler, A. Love and adulthood in American culture. In J.J. Smelser and E. H. Erickson (Eds.), *Themes of love and work in adulthood.* Cambridge: Howard University Press, 1980, 120-150.

Wachowiak, D., and Bragg, H. Open marriage and marital adjustment. *Journal of Marriage and the Family,* 1980, 42, 57-62.

Walen, S. Cognitive factors in sexual behavior. *Journal of Sex and Marital Therapy.* 1980, 6, 87-101.

Walster, E., Traupmann, J., and Walster, W. Equity and extramarital sexuality. *Archives of Sexual Behavior,* 1978, 7, 127-142.

Westoff, C. F., and Ryder, N. B. *The contraceptive revolution.* Princeton, NJ: Princeton University Press, 1977.

Wolfe, L. The sexual profile of that cosmopolitan girl. *Cosmopolitan,* September 1980, 254-265.

Zilbergeld, B. *Male sexuality.* Boston: Little Brown, 1978.

3

Measuring the Process of Fertility Decision-Making

Linda J. Beckman

Decisions made by couples regarding the use of contraception and the planning and spacing of children can be conceptualized as intervening variables in a dynamic multistage process. This sequential process involves the influences of demographic, developmental, biological, psychological, and social-psychological factors on the formation and stability of preferences, intentions, and decisions regarding fertility and contraception, and the intervening effects of these fertility decision variables upon subsequent desires, decisions, and fertility outcomes. Among couples in all but the most transient of relationships, males as well as females are involved in this process of preference formation and decision-making.

That fertility decision-making frequently is sequential in nature is self-evident, but the exact nature of this sequential process remains a matter of controversy. Some contend that various sequences or subsequences of events occur in determination of fertility decisions (for example, Hass, 1974; Miller and Godwin, 1977). Hass (1974) has distinguished three possible stages of fertility decisions: the preconception stage, the pregnancy stage, and the postnatal stage. At each of these stages the fertility decision to be made differs (for example, "shall I use contraception?" versus "Shall I have an abortion?"), as does the action undertaken to prevent or facilitate fertility and the probable fertility outcome. Other researchers also assume that couples and individuals pass through various stages before reaching a decision regarding intrastage events, such as remaining childless (Veevers, 1973), obtaining an abortion (Diamond et al., 1973; Rosen, 1976), or bearing an unwanted child (Freedman and Berelson, 1976).

Although prior stages and decisions influence current fertility decision-making, it frequently is assumed, as in the Hass model, that the decision made at one time point involves only the current birth rather than long-term fertility planning. However, my own data, indicating that about 30 percent of young married couples in Los Angeles County reported a joint decision regarding *total* number of children (Beckman, 1979), suggest that the preconception decision may involve total family size as well as the next child. These data also show that a reassessment of previous decisions frequently occurs as a result of a fertility outcome, particularly the birth of a first child.

Fertility decisions may follow various patterns and may involve a long- or short-term time frame. For instance, some persons only decide not to have a child "now", while others decide they want no more children. Some couples drift into parenthood without making any conscious decision, while others conscientiously plan the timing of the first birth. Some partners modify their preferences and decisions as a result of their parenthood experiences, while others do not. Outside of a few notable exceptions (see Neal and Groat, 1980), these different decision-making styles have not been adequately studied to date.

As implied above, different degrees of fertility decision-making may occur. Of the couples in my sample, 34 percent disagreed about whether they had made certain pre-conception fertility decisions. Such lack of congruence in spouses' responses partly may be due to varying notions of what a "decision" is. For some people a general discussion and agreement about an issue may indicate a decision ("We both felt it would be all right if we had another child sometime"), whereas for others such a statement is associated with uncertainty. For the second group a decision may involve a definite verbal commitment to a plan of action ("We decided that after my husband finishes school next year, I will try to get pregnant"). It is evident, however, that a fertility decision is not an all-or-nothing phenomenon — that decisions vary in type, style, the strength with which they are held and adhered to, and the degree to which they are explicit rather than implicit.

The questions of what aspects of fertility decision-making to study and how they should be studied remain open. For example, at which time points should the process be measured? Which variables or constructs should be measured? Which measurement techniques should be used to examine how fertility decisions are made (if indeed they are) and how such decisions influence fertility outcomes?

The questions posed are complex and cannot be solved by a simple set of guidelines. The issues and problems surrounding each of these questions, however, can be identified, and this is the major purpose of the remainder of this chapter.

WHAT TO MEASURE?

Social scientists usually want to understand what influences the decision-making process and how fertility preferences and decisions are themselves related to actual fertility. As our measurement techniques have become more sophisticated, researchers have increasingly become interested in explicating causal relationships among sets of variables rather than simply determining which of several simultaneously considered nonfertility varables are related to fertility decision-making. In this endeavor, fertility decision-making can be conceptualized as a intervening variable that illuminates the effects of demographic, psychological, and social variables upon fertility-related behaviors and outcomes.

Fertility Decisions and Outcomes

The question of what specific variables should be measured within the broad spectrum of what can be called fertility choice and decision variables, of course, depends on the aims of one's research. A variety of fertility-decision-related variables exists — desires, intentions, decisions, behaviors. These types of variables may be thought of as occupying a continuum in terms of distance from a fertility outcome, or composing a specified sequence of the substages that leads to a fertility outcome. A desire or intention indicates an individual-level attitudinal variable, while a decision indicates a couple-based process.

When studying intentions or decisions, actual fertility outcomes (such as whether an intention to have a child will result in a pregnancy within two years) or fertility behaviors (such as whether the couple will discontinue use of contraception) are usually the final dependent variables of choice. Most frequently, however, the intention or decision itself is the final variable considered, because study of some fertility events (such as a pregnancy or live birth) requires costly longitudinal designs or must use methodologically suspect retrospective information regarding past desires, decisions, and intentions (Kiesler, 1977). One important facet of social-psychological research investigates the intention-behavior relationship and the particular variables influencing the strength of this relationship (see Davidson and Jaccard, 1979; Kar and Talbot, 1980).

Although the temporal periods during which desires, preferences, or decisions are measured, as well as the selection of fertility variables themselves, depend on the specific purpose of the research, conceptualization of fertility decision-making as a couple-based process that occurs over time extends the range of factors that might be measured. In addition to type and strength of individual desires and intentions, the types, strategies, strength, and explicitness of decisions made by couples can be measured. Couple-based variables measured at various stages of the family-building cycle can include congruence between the reported decisions, patterns of agreement regarding fertility preferences, accuracy of perception regarding the other's fertility preferences (and thus the explicitness of disagreements), and strategies used for resolution of disagreements regarding individual preferences. Procedures for dealing with couple responses are discussed later.

Some of these measures have been examined in previous research (see Beckman, 1979; Loscuito et al., 1978; Mellinger et al., 1977; Miller, 1980). While the details of these studies will not be discussed here, these researchers do suggest variables that might be important in future studies.

One caveat regarding selection of fertility variables for study is that the more specific the action and the more limited the time period, generally the greater the relationship among antecedent variables, fertility intentions, and fertility outcomes (Davidson and Jaccard, 1979; Fisbein and Ajzen, 1975). Therefore, the less global the fertility-related outcome, the more likely the study is to produce meaningful and significant results. Thus, it usually is better to investigate current use of specific methods of contraception than it is to determine ever-use. Similarly, for most purposes, intention to have a

child within the next two years is probably _____
number of children desired.

Independent Variables

In addition to considering the stability of pr_
fertility and the effects of fertility preferences, dec.
and outcomes upon subsequent fertility variables, ___s of
fertility decision-making attempt to examine sets o_ __ables believed to influence fertility decisions, behaviors, or outcomes. Such
antecedent indepent variables include the following categories:

(1) demographic and background, such as age, age at marriage, religion, ethnicity, socioeconomic status, divorce, and remarriage;

(2) psychological traits, such as locus of control, sex role traditionalism, alienation, and personal efficacy;

(3) attitudinal, such as perceived values of children, motivations regarding parenthood, knowledge and acceptability of birth planning,
attitudes regarding conception, sexuality, and abortion;

(4) biological, such as subfecundity, sterility;

(5) social-psychological, such as power in the family, openness of
communication, social support from others; and

(6) developmental, such as age of children, life-cycle stage, own
socialization experiences.

Subsequent chapters explore various sets of variables outlined
above.

Any or all of the above categories can be built into a model of the
fertility decision process, but, given the present perspective, the most
interesting set is the social-psychological, because only these factors
build on the interpersonal nature of the decision process. Many are
unique to a decision-making model, whereas the other sets of variables apply equally well to a model that only examines intentions of
one person, generally the female partner.

MEASUREMENT PROBLEMS AND TECHNIQUES

My recommendations regarding measurement techniques are
based on problems that frequently arise due to the nature of fertility
variables and the decision process. First, the process being meas-

if there is only one outcome variable of fertility choice or on, is a complex, fluid, and dynamic one. In order to study or tempt to model such a process, even using only a few antecedent variables, a multivariate analysis is appropriate. Although this approach may be as simple as standard multiple regression, it is likely that more complex structural equation models that specify causal linkages among independent and dependent variables (Duncan, 1975; Heise, 1975; Joreskog and Sorbom, 1979) are required.

A second methodological problem is that fertility variables are usually discrete rather than continuous in nature. For instance, we study whether a couple has or has not made a decision to have a child in the next two years, or whether a couple is or is not using a particular method of contraception. Even when our intervening or outcome variables approach being continuous (for example, the total number of children a person intends or has), the shape of the distribution rarely approaches normality but rather is highly skewed. Although sometimes nothing can be done about the nature of these variables, an important caution is in order. Most of our current multivariate statistical techniques based on assumptions regarding multivariate normal distributions and frequently uncorrelated error variance may not be equal to the task of handling such discrete variables, particularly when in combination with continuous antecedent or intervening variables.[1] We assume these techniques are robust but frequently do not know the effects of departures from assumptions such as multivariate normality. Furthermore, there appears to be no current methodology that handles all the other limitations of variables in fertility models and also can completely successfully deal with the categorical nature of fertility variables. Therefore, whenever possible, it is desirable to use measurement methods that produce variables that approach a continuum.

Third, even when individual responses are considered, although reporting of some fertility variables (such as number of living children) may not be subject to much measurement error, other variables (such as motivations for parenthood) may be characterized by significant measurement error. Furthermore, the methodology most often used in social science research to collect fertility-related information, survey questionnaires, contains several sources of measurement error, including subject forgetting, rationalization, or distortion; ceiling or floor effects; incorrect recording of the data by interviewers; and various yea-saying or social desirability biases. Such measurement error, random and nonrandom, can be taken into account in some of the measurement models employed (Alwin and Jackson, 1980). If such error is not taken into account, it is likely that significant relationships between constructs will be attenuated (Heise, 1969) and reliability and stability of constructs may be incorrectly estimated (Wheaton et al., 1977).

Finally, when intentions or decisions are measured, the investigator must deal with the difficult and sometimes distressing problems of what to do with responses, often differing responses, from two separate people. Although a standard procedure has been simply to average couple responses, if indeed the couple rather than the individual is the unit of analysis, their joint pattern of response must be considered. It is necessary to decide whether two persons' responses are multiple indicators of the same reality, such as number of times had sexual intercourse in last week, or separate indicators of different realities, such as number of children desired by each spouse (Thompson, 1980). It may also be possible in cases of disagreement to determine which spouse is likely to be the more accurate reporter of an action. For instance, in cases of disagreement, I decided to use wife's response regarding birth control rather than husband's response, because the great majority of couples used female-controlled methods such as the Pill and the IUD, and use/nonuse of contraception may have more severe consequences for women in terms of the subsequent impact of a conception or birth.

In instances where there is no particular reason to believe one gender's response to be more accurate or valid, two strategies appear appropriate. First, when responses are assumed to measure the same entity or construct, the lack of reliability of spouses' responses may be treated as a fact in its own right. In the type of model I will be discussing later, it is possible to treat these responses as multiple indicators of the *same* construct (for example, relative power in the dyad). Such an approach allows disagreements between husbands and wives to be treated as measurement error using factor-analytic methods. .

The second approach is to use degree of concurrence (or agreement) and accuracy of perception as intervening variables. Concurrence measures the extent to which persons hold similar perceptions, knowledge, or attitudes on an issue (such as the number of children to have). It can be defined as degree of independent agreement of both members of a couple. Such agreement may be based on commonly

shared socialization experiences leading to internalization or acceptance of norms defining appropriate fertility behavior (Hollerbach,
1980), or on chance. In the case of fertility decisions, concurrence
between spouses regarding types and styles of joint decisions may be
influenced by communication styles and patterns and family power,
rather than by unspoken but shared norms regarding fertility.
Furthermore, techniques have been developed that purport to distinguish agreements based on chance from mutually recognized agreement (Coombs and Fernandez, 1978; Yaukey et al., 1967).

Accuracy of perception is the degree to which one spouse can
accurately predict the responses of the other. It can be measured by
the correlation or percentage of agreement between the responses of
one spouse and the predictions of the second spouse about the first
spouse's responses.

The above four interrelated measurement problems — discrete
variables, measurement error, couple responses, and complex processes — are inherent in all but very simple studies of the fertility
decision-making process, and they lead to problems regarding reliability and validity of data. For instance, large amounts of random
measurement error are considered synonomous with unreliability
(Heise, 1969; Wiley and Wiley, 1970). Couple data, if averaged, may
yield invalid and incomplete information. Discrete variables with
extreme distributions may provide distorted results in multivariate
analysis. On the other hand, if complex real-world processes are
analyzed using simplistic techniques, it is unlikely that a gain in
knowledge regarding fertility processes will occur.

The best class of analytic techniques to deal with these types of
measurement problems seem to be a group of structural equation
models that do not assume perfect measurement of each variable
(Alwin and Jackson, 1980; Bentler, 1980; Bielby et al., 1976; Blalock,
1970; Hannan et al., 1974; Hauser and Goldberger, 1971; Joreskog,
1973; Joreskog and Sorbom, 1979; Wheaton et al., 1977). Most of these
models can be estimated within the framework of the Joreskog and
Sorbom (1978) approach for analysis of linear structural relationships
by the method of maximum likelihood (LISREL), although other
solutions, not based on maximum likelihood, also exist (see Wold,
1979).

In the LISREL formulation, two types of models are used. The
measurement model specifies the measurement of latent variables (or
hypothetical constructs) in terms of observed variables. It is used to

estimate the measurement properties — that is, reliabilities and validities — of the observed variables. The structural equation model is used to specify causal relationships among latent variables, the strength of causal effects, and the amount of unexplained variance (Joreskog and Sorbom, 1978).

The strength of the LISREL approach is its ability to deal with measurement error through estimation of unobserved variables based on multiple indicators. If all variables in a fertility decision-making model are assumed to be perfectly measured (a very unlikely occurrence) and causal relationships are assumed to be recursive (the variables are ordered in such a way that all causal arrows go only in one direction and reciprocal causation does not occur), path analysis using least squares multiple regression is simpler to use. If simultaneous reciprocal causation (that is, X influences Y *and* Y influences X) is thought to occur among perfectly measured constructs, multiple regression, using two-stage least squares, may be employed (see Waite and Stolzenberg, 1976). Also, LISREL assumes linearity of relationships and cannot adequately deal with interactions among variables.

For the reader who understands the basics of multiple regression analysis, some further explanation may be useful. Least squares regression minimizes the sum of squares between the observed and estimated parameters; that is, it minimizes the error variance. This has the effect of estimating regression coefficients with the lowest possible variance. But such estimated parameters are likely to be biased, usually downwardly, because of measurement error; that is, an incorrect parameter is likely to be estimated quite precisely. Correcting a regression coefficient for attenuation frequently produces a stronger relationship between structural parameters but this is not inevitably true.

Attenuated estimates are likely in structural equation models when measurement error exists or when significant variables are omitted. In contrast with least squares regression, Joreskog's model and others (most using maximum likelihood) that estimate measurement error eliminate some bias in estimated parameters, but at the expense of decreased precision; that is, they should produce estimated scores closer to the true score but at the same time have greater variance (Joreskog, 1980).

Frequently the effects of omitted variables can be considered in such models through specification of correlated disturbance terms or correlations between exogenous variables and disturbance terms. Correlated measurement error terms frequently are used to specify nonrandom "method" sources of measurement error.

I hope the above discussion has given the reader some idea of the difficulties involved in measuring the determinants and characteristics of the fertility decision process. In the next section I would like to discuss further the types of problems an investigator must solve when studying fertility variables, using an example from my own research in progress.

TESTING OF FERTILITY DECISION-MAKING MODELS

My colleagues and I were interested in both individual and couple variables. On the level of the individual, we studied how background variables affected motivations and attitudes regarding parenthood, employment, and women's roles and how these motivations subsequently affected fertility desires and intentions. On the couple level, our interest was in couple interaction, communication, and power and their effects on joint decisions and fertility outcomes as well as individual intentions.

The models, described in Figures 3.1 and 3.2, concentrate on the preconception phase of fertility decision-making among married couples. Originally, a joint model included all variables — husband, wife, and couple — but the limitations of analytic techniques were such that it was essential that the larger model, which contained about 25 latent and over 50 observed variables, be subdivided into three smaller chunks.

Operationalization of Variables

Background and demographic variables originally examined included age, age at marriage, socioeconomic status, and religion and ethnicity (both of which, because of their categorical, nature had been coded as dummy varibles).[2] These demographic variables were portrayed as *exogenous* variables that were not causally affected by other variables to the right of them, as shown in Figures 3.1 and 3.2. The only imperfectly measured exogenous construct was socio-

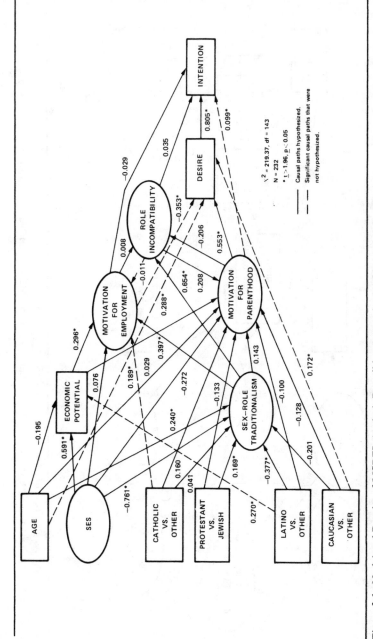

Figure 3.1 Model and Results of LISREL Analysis Describing Antecedents of Intention for Wives

NOTE: LISREL analysis limited to *married* wives.

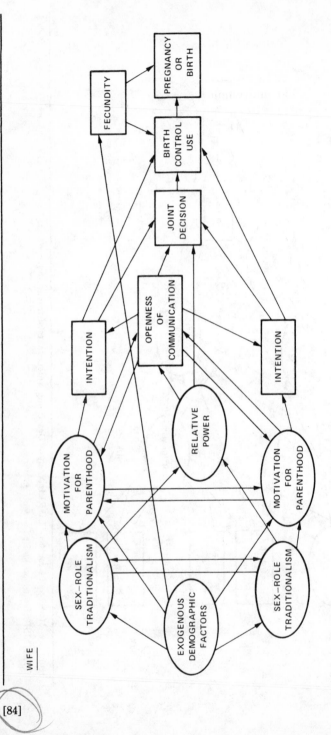

Figure 3.2 Joint Couple Model of Antecedents of Fertility

NOTE: Endogenous employment-related variables are omitted from the model. Correlated error terms also are not included.

economic status, which was indicated by own income, own education, and own socioeconomic status (based on the Duncan SEI).

Individual-level endogenous variables originally included motivation for parenthood and employment, sex role traditionalism, economic potential, current employment status, perceived role incompatibility, and fertility desires and intentions regarding a child in the next two years. For men, attitude toward wife's employment was substituted for perceived role incompatibility. Desire was a dichotomous yes-no variable, while intention was based on the degree of certainty that one would or would not have a child in the next two years (with values ranging from -7, "definitely will not have a child," to $+7$, "definitely will have"). The latent constructs measured by multiple indicators included motivation for parenthood, motivation for employment, perceived role incompatibility, and attitude toward wife's work. For instance, motivation toward parenthood was composed of three observed variables: the sum of the satisfactions of parenthood, the sum of the costs of parenthood, and a summary index of perceived normative influence.

Couple-marital dyad-level variables included relative power of spouses, measured in terms of both general and specific decision-making factors and the husbands' and wives' relative resources; openness of communication between spouses regarding fertility, birth control, and sexuality; joint decision patterns regarding a child in the next two years (coded as $1 = $ decide yes, $2 = $ conflicted or uncertain, and $3 = $ decide no); consistency of contraception use over an 18-20-month period (coded as consistent or inconsistent); and presence or absence of an intervening birth or pregnancy during this same period.

Among the couple variables, openness of communication and relative power are conceptualized as latent constructs. Couple communication consisted of two wife and two husband indices. For each spouse, openness of fertility-specific discussion was rated separately for self and for spouse. Relative power was measured by four wife and four husband variables. For each spouse, the observed variables were the sum of five fertility-related decision items (such as when to have the next child), with each decision weighted by its importance and higher scores indicating more wife power; sum of the ratings of 11 other decisions (such as where to go on vacation), each weighted by importance; perceived relative resources of self minus spouse, based on a 20-item self-administered semantic differential rating of attributes of self and an identical rating of spouse; and finally, a summary index of the relative extent to which spouses showed four behaviors — arguing in front of someone else, threatening to leave, being stubborn, hitting or throwing things — that may be thought of as coercive and may provide an indication of commitment to the relationship.

In Figures 3.1 and 3.2, when a latent (unobserved) variable is assumed to be perfectly measured by one observed variable, it is indicated by a rectangle, whereas a latent variable assumed to include measurement error is indicated by an ellipse. The variables indicated as being perfectly measured (for example, desire), obviously contain some measurement error, but because only one observed measure of these variables was available and its reliability could not be estimated, such error could not be taken into account.

The Model

The theoretical model expounded is based on the premise that, in general, sociodemographic characteristics affect fertility intentions, decisions, and outcomes only indirectly, through their effects on both the cognitive and the affective components of attitudes (that is, beliefs and motivations) and the opportunity costs of children (measured by economic potential). Fertility desires, intentions, and decisions are conceptualized as intervening variables in the process by which exogenous sociodemographic variables affect fertility behaviors and outcomes. In this complex sequential process, internalized motivations affect desires, which, in turn, are translated into intentions regarding childbearing. Intentions influence joint decisions and, depending on the joint decision process, may directly or indirectly affect patterns of contraception and fertility outcomes. Fertility intentions may be conceptualized as the end product of individual decision-making, while decisions are the end result of couple communication and decision-making, directly affecting contraception use and, thus, fertility outcomes.

Based on my own previous research (Beckman, 1979), it was hypothesized that desires and intentions that represent conceptually distinct dimensions of fertility attitudes are differently affected by other attitudinal factors. As shown by the solid lines in Figure 3.1, among women intention is hypothesized to be indirectly influenced by motivation for parenthood and directly influenced by motivation for alternative roles, such as employment, and by perceived incompatibility between parenthood and these other roles. Desire for a child, in contrast, is affected only by motivation for parenthood. The higher the motivation for employment and the greater the perceived incompatibility of employment and parenthood, the greater the negative effect on birth intentions.

Among men a slightly different model from that shown in Figure 3.1 is believed to apply. Perceived role incompatibility is omitted and attitude toward wife's employment substituted. Both attitude toward wife's employment and motivation for own employment are hypothesized directly to affect birth intentions, and attitude toward wife's employment is thought to have reciprocal effects with motivation for parenthood.

The economic opportunity costs of children, measured by the proxy variable, economic potential, also are hypothesized to influence intentions of both spouses through their effects on motivations for both employment and parenthood. Most general sex role attitudes (that is, sex role traditionalism) are causally connected to specific attitudes and motivations regarding own employment (for women), wife's employment (for husbands), and parenthood.

The joint decision is affected by the couple-level variables of communication in the marital dyad and relative power of spouses. It was tentatively assumed (see Figure 3.2) that openness of couple communication affected fertility decisions (or the lack thereof) in one of two ways. First, communication may lead directly to decision. Second, communication can lead to change in the intentions of one or both spouses; this may occur either directly or through the effects of communication on motivation for parenthood. Relative power of spouses is primarily important when couples do not initially agree regarding fertility preferences. In cases of disagreement, the final decision may directly depend on the relative power of the spouses. Relative power also may affect openness of communication, which, in turn, affects the joint decision made.

One member of a couple may make a unilateral and/or surreptitious decision regarding parenthood, but usually in stable couple relationships fertility regulation is not based on such decisions. Open unilateral decisions, however, may occur when one spouse has much greater power than the other. Surreptitious (and, by definition, unilateral) decisions may occur when a spouse with low observed power, usually the wife, feels a strong need to control the fertility outcome. The joint decision itself, of necessity, is characterized in the present model as a categorical variable, based on whether both spouses report a decision has been made and what the decision is. In cases of nondecision, couple conflict regarding preferences is distinguished from differing perceptions regarding what constitutes a decision.

Methods

Data are based upon a longitudinal study of a sample of 507 young couples residing in Los Angeles County. The sample was limited to legally married couples, with wife aged 18 to 34. The majority of the sample was drawn from county birth and marriage records. However, 30.6 percent were identified through a modified snowballing technique: Respondents in the first group were asked to identify neighbors or friends who were eligible for the study; 232 of the couples (the married group) had recently married for the first time and had no children; 275 couples (the babied group) had recently had their first child.

Each spouse separately participated in two interviews, the first approximately six months after the event (first marriage or first birth) and the second approximately twenty months after the initial interview. The instruments measured reported fertility decisions and preferences, perceived rewards and costs of parenthood, perceptions of characteristics associated with wife's employment, decision-making, power and communication in the marital dyad, use of contraception, economic factors, and other demographic information.

Analytic Procedures Used

The use of LISREL frequently requires that less complex techniques be employed antecedent to its own use. A first step for each of the three models was to obtain start values for use with the LISREL computer program (Joreskog and Sorbom, 1978). Because maximum likelihood procedures involve an iterative process by which sample parameters are adjusted until the likelihood of sample values approaching theoretical values is maximized, the LISREL program needs start values for estimated parameters at which to begin its iterations. The further away these start values are from the final values for a parameter, the more unlikely it is that the program will reach a satisfactory solution. Therefore, it is desirable to compute a standard path analysis (using least squares multiple regression) to estimate start values for causal relationships, and, when latent variables are composed of several observed variables, to use factor analysis to estimate start values for measurement models.

For all three models, maximum likelihood factor analysis was used to obtain factor loadings. Standardized path coefficients were then computed, using factor scores to estimate latent variables. In all analyses, separate start values were obtained for the married and the babied samples, because it was suspected that certain structural relationships may have differing strengths, depending on a couples' place in the family-building process.

One problem evident in these data was the redundancy of some of the variables in the models. This redundancy frequently gives rise to statistical problems regarding multicolinearity — the existence of high intercorrelations among a set of independent variables, which can lead to highly misleading and attenuated regression coefficients for the entire set and reduced sampling stability (Cohen and Cohen, 1975).

Among observed variables deleted were age at marriage, highly redundant with current age; current employment status, highly redundant with economic potential; and socioeconomic status. The latent variable, economic potential, was revised to exclude measures of present status (that is, amount worked since marriage, amount paid last week), which were highly correlated with one of the indices of SES, own income. Economic potential was redefined as *gain* in economic potential, operationalized by estimated income at age 50 minus own current income, to allow examination of economic potential net of the effects of current income. This measure, however, has the disadvantage of not allowing estimation of measurement error.

Other problems regarding the two latent economic variables involved missing data. As expected, income was the observed variable on which the greatest percent of people failed to provide information. In the present data, 13.6 percent of the sample did not provide current yearly income, and 16.2 percent did not state their income for the last week worked. In order to salvage the construct "socioeconomic class" as originally defined, it was necessary to estimate missing values for income by regressing own income on the best linear combination of two available variables and then using the equation obtained to estimate missing values.[3] Other improved methods for dealing with missing data on panel studies have recently been described by Marini et al. (1980).

Testing the Models

Once preliminary analyses had been run, the following steps were taken to test the model using LISREL. In some cases, problems described above occurred and were resolved during these steps rather than preceding them. First, the measurement model was assessed separately for each latent variable. Next, causal paths were added between variables, first for the endogenous variables (that is, those affected by other variables in the model) and next for exogenous variables. Finally, in cases of presumed reciprocal causality, a second arrow was added between two variables to indicate bidirectional causality. In some cases, paths were added (or omitted) when alternative, theoretically based specifications appeared to fit the data better than the original model. The three models were examined for babieds and marrieds separately. Sometimes when a model had been built for one group, several steps in the above procedure could be short-circuited for the second group.

The above procedure is costly in terms of computer and programmer time. Since one does not usually start with a completed model, the process of building up a model may require a large number of computer runs using the LISREL program; even though the groundwork for finding start values has been completed, 15-40 runs per group is not unusual with a complex model. Particularly in cases where the program does not converge because of poor start values, inadequate data, or a misspecified model, this process can be very expensive.

Although I discuss building up a model, it is essential that the reader understand that in any model-testing (using path analysis, structural equation models, or structural equation models plus measurement models), it is imperative that the investigator begin with a sound theoretical conceptualization to be tested or a few alternative models to be compared. With several variables, a large variety of models is possible, and these methods should not be used as fishing expeditions to determine which of a large number of possible alternatives is best. They can test whether a model is plausible or better than another clearly specified causal model, given the interrelationship among variables (the correlation or covariance matrix), but one must decide whether one's model is theoretically defensible.

The more complex the statistical technique, the more critical it is that the investigator begin with a clearly specified model. If not, it is very likely that results will be expensive, unmeaningful, and/or form the basis of incorrect interpretations.

Married Wives

Given the limited scope of this chapter, it is impossible to discuss all three models for each of two groups (Some of these models are not yet completely analyzed.) However, I would like to discuss the final wife model of the married group, which is shown in Figure 3.1, to provide an example of what kind of information can be gleaned and relationships explicated by combining causal and measurement models. Since the extent of measurement error is not indicated in Figure 3.1, a few comments should be made regarding it. Measurement error of the individual observed variables was high, particularly for the constructs of motivation for parenthood, motivation for employment, and role incompatibility, suggesting that the structural coefficients would have been attenuated had not such error been taken into account. Generally, however, little intercorrelated measurement error was found in the present data set, indicating, perhaps, lack of method effects.

Figure 3.1 shows standardized regression coefficients (betas and gammas in LISREL terminology) that, wherever possible, have been corrected for measurement error. All paths specified in the original model (the solid lines in Figure 3.1) have been retained, and new paths found to be statistically significant (the dashed lines in Figure 3.1) have been added. Examination of Figure 3.1 reveals instances where causal relationships or the lack thereof specified by the original model were not upheld. (It should be noted that the chi square to degrees of freedom ratio for goodness of fit in Figure 3.1 of 1.5 [219.37/143] indicates that even the revised model does not reproduce the original correlation matrix extremely well. A 1.0 ratio would indicate a very good fit.)

It was assumed that exogenous sociodemographic characteristics affect fertility intentions only through their indirect effects on motivations and beliefs (regarding sex roles or economic potential). As predicted, background variables had no direct effects on intentions, but contrary to prediction there were two direct links to desire for a child in the next two years: age and being Caucasian both positively affected desire. Also, several predicted paths from background variables to attitudes and motivations were not upheld (as indicated by insignificant path coefficients in Figure 3.1).

It also was predicted that desire would be directly influenced only by motivation for parenthood, while in fact desire also was found to be a significant consequence of motivation for employment and demographic factors. Furthermore, no direct path between motivation for parenthood and intention was included in the original model in Figure 3.1, while a direct link was hypothesized between motivation for employment and intention. The final results obtained, however, were the opposite of those specified in the theoretical model. Motivation for parenthood had a small but statistically significant direct effect on intention, as well as a larger indirect effect through desire. Motivation for employment appeared to affect intention neither directly nor through role incompatibility; its effects on intention seem primarily to be via its negative relationship with desire.

These results may suggest a preconscious dimension of motivation for parenthood which directly influences intention rather than being mediated by conscious preference. Motivation for the alternative role of employment appears directly to influence preference for children rather than serving as a construct mediating between desire and intention. Role incompatibility, which was hypothesized to be a key variable in the model, was strongly positively influenced by sex role traditionalism. Role incompatibility had *no* significant effects on any endogenous variables. On the other hand, both sex role traditionalism and economic potential strongly affected motivation for employment. Their causal links to motivation for parenthood, although in the predicted direction, were not significant.

Finally, ethnicity and religion frequently influenced sex role and motivational variables in unexpected ways. Latinos reported expecting greater gain in economic potential than did other ethnic groups, and Caucasians were more rather than less likely than other groups to desire a child in the next two years. Also, Catholic women reported higher motivation for employment (as did Latinos, indirectly, through economic potential) than did the other sociodemographic groups. At the same time, however Catholic women also reported somewhat greater motivation for parenthood. These results may indicate, within our relatively well-educated sample, the presence of a subgroup of Latino Catholic women who perceive themselves as nontraditional and highly motivated toward career, yet who also evidence high motivation for parenthood.

CONCLUSION

This chapter has considered measurement problems that arise because of the sequential and complex nature of the fertility decision-making process. Decisions regarding fertility may vary in type, style, strength, and explicitness. A broad range of fertility preference, decision, and outcome variables are available to be measured, as are antecedent independent variables that measure psychological, or biological dimensions. Specific measurement problems discussed include couple responses, discrete variables, measurement error in survey data, and complex processes. A class of analytic techniques based on maximum likelihood that can deal with most, but not all, of these measurement problems was described, and an example was presented from my own work. The use of less complex regression and factor techniques prior to employing LISREL, and the process of building up and testing a model, was broadly described. It is important that the investigator start with a clearly specified theoretical conceptualization or a few alternative models to be compared.

NOTES

1. There are specific techniques for analyzing categorical data, such as log-linear analyses, logistic regression, and logit and probit analysis, (see Benedetti and Brown, 1976; Bishop et al., 1975; Cox, 1970).

2. As described later in this chapter, employment status and age at marriage were later deleted because of their redundancy with other variables.

3. The two variables generally used were percentage of income from husband and a categorical question regarding income above or below $10,000. Alternative estimators used when these variables were also missing were the Duncan SEI and education. In this procedure it is not inappropriate to use other observed variables within a construct as missing value estimators.

REFERENCES

Alwin, D. F., and Jackson, D. J. Measurement models for response errors in surveys: Issues and applications. In K. F. Schuessler (Ed.), *Sociological methodology.* San Francisco: Jossey-Bass, 1980.

Beckman, L. J. *The process of couples' fertility decision-making.* Paper presented at the Family Planning, Contraception, and Abortion Symposium of the American Psychological Association meetings, New York, September 1979.

Benedetti, J. K., and Brown, M. B. Alternate methods of building log-linear models. *Proceedings of the 9th International Biometric Conference,* 1976, 2, 209-227.

Bentler, P. M. Multivariate analysis with latent variables: Causal modeling. *Annual Review of Psychology,* 1980, 31, 419-456.

Bielby, W. T., Hauser, R. M., and Featherman, D. L. Response errors of non-black males in models of the stratification process. *American Journal of Sociology,* 1976, 82, 1242-1288.

Bishop, Y. M. M., Feinberg, S. E., and Holland, P. W. *Discrete multivariate analysis: Theory and practice.* Cambridge, MA: MIT Press, 1975.

Blalock, H. M., Jr. Estimating measurement error using multiple indicators and several points in time. *American Sociological Review,* 1970, 35, 101-111.

Cohen, J., and Cohen P. *Applied multiple regression/correlation analysis for the behavioral sciences.* Hillsdale, NJ: Lawrence Erlbaum Associates, 1975.

Coombs, L. C., and Fernandez, D. Husband-wife agreement about reproductive goals. *Demography,* 1978, 15(1), 57-73.

Cox, D. R. *The analysis of binary data.* London: Methuen, 1970.

Davidson, A. R., and Jaccard, J. J. Variables that moderate the attitude-behavior relation: Results of a longitudinal survey. *Journal of Personality and Social Psychology,* 1979, 37(8), 364-376.

Diamond, M., Steinhoff, P. G., Palmore, J. A., and Smith, R. G. Sexuality, birth control, and abortion; A decision-making sequence, *Journal of Biosocial Science,* 1973, 5, 346-361.

Duncan, O. D. *Introduction to structural equation models.* New York: Academic Press, 1975.

Fishbein, M., and Ajzen, S. *Belief, attitude, intention, and behavior: An introduction to theory and research.* Reading, MA: Addison-Wesley, 1975.

Freedman, R., and Berelson, B. The record of family planning programs. *Studies on Family Planning,* 1976, 7(1), 1-40.

Hannan, M. T., Rubenson, R., and Warren, J. T. The causal approach to measurement error in panel analysis: Some further contingencies. In H. M. Blalock, Jr. (Ed.), *Measurement in the social sciences: Theories and strategies.* Chicago: Aldine, 1974.

Hass, P. H. Wanted and unwanted pregnancies: A fertility decision-making model. *Journal of Social Issues,* 1974, 30(4), 125-165.

Hauser, R. M., and Goldberger, A. S. The treatment of unobservable variables in path analysis. In H. L. Castner (Ed.), *Sociological methodology.* San Francisco: Jossey-Bass, 1971.

Heise, D. R. Separating reliability and stability in test-retest correlation. *American Sociological Review,* 1969, 34, 94-101.

Heise, D. R. *Causal analysis.* New York: Wiley, 1975.

Hollerbach, P. E. Power in families, communication, and fertility decision-making. *Population and Environment: Behavioral and Social Issues,* 1980, 3(2), 146-194.

Joreskog, K. G. A general method for estimating a linear structural equation system. In A. G. Goldberger and O. D. Duncan (Eds.), *Structural equation models in the social sciences.* New York: Seminar, 1973.

Joreskog, K. G. Lecture presented at the Linear Structural Relationships and Factor Analysis Professional Development Training Seminar, Department of Education, University of Chicago, September 1980.

Joreskog, K. G. and Sorbom, D. *LISREL IV – A general computer program for estimation of a linear structural equation system by maximum likelihood methods.* Chicago: National Educational Resources, 1978.

Joreskog, K. G., and Sorbom, D. *Advances in factor analysis and structural equation models.* Cambridge, MA: Abt, 1979.

Kar, S. B., and Talbot, J. M. Attitudinal and non-attitudinal determinants of contraception: A cross-cultural study. *Studies in Family Planning,* 1980, 11(2), 51-64.

Kiesler, S. B. Post hoc justification of family size. *Sociometry,* 1977, 40(1), 59-67.

LoScuito, L., Peterson, J., and Ausetts, M. A. *Fertility-related decision-making among married couples.* Unpublished manuscript, Institute for Survey Research, Temple University, 1978.

Marini, M. M., Olsen, A. R., and Ruben, D. B. Maximum likelihood estimation in panel studies with missing data. In K. F. Schuessler (Ed.), *Sociological methodology*. San Francisco: Jossey-Bass, 1980.

Mellinger, G., Muller, K., and Tiktinsky, M. *Motivational conflict and couple fertility decisions*. Report of preliminary results prepared for NICHD (R01 HD09246) by the Institute for Research in Social Behavior, Berkeley, Ca., 1977.

Miller, W. B. *The psychology of reproduction*. Final report to the Center for Population Research, NICHD(N01-HD-82831), by the American Institutes for Research, Palo Alto, California, 1980.

Miller, W. B., and Godwin, R. K. *Psyche and Demos: Individual psychology and the issues of population*. New York: Oxford University Press, 1977.

Neal, A. G., and Groat, H. T. Fertility decision-making, unintended births, and the social drift hypothesis: A longitudinal study. *Population and Environment: Behavioral and Social Issues*, 1980, 3(3/4), 210-220.

Rosen R. A. *Decision-making on unplanned problem pregnancies*. Final report, Department of Sociology, Wayne State University, Detroit, 1976.

Thomson, E. *Remarks regarding multi-component units of analysis*. Paper presented at Eighth Annual Workshop on Phychosocial Factors in Population Research, Denver, Colorado, April 1980.

Veevers, J. E. Voluntary childless wives: An exploratory study. *Sociology and Social Research*, 1973, 57(3), 356-366.

Waite, L. J. and Stolzenberg, R. M. Intended childbearing and labor force participation of young women: Insights from nonrecursive models. *American Sociological Review*, 1976, 41, 235-252.

Wheaton, B., Muthen, B., Alwin, D. F. and Summers, G. F. Assessing reliability and stability in panel models. In D. R. Heise (Ed.), *Sociological methodology*. San Francisco: Jossey-Bass, 1977.

Wiley, D. E., and Wiley, J. A. The estimation of measurement error in panel data. *American Sociological Review*, 1970, 35, 112-117.

Wold, H. Model construction and evaluation when theoretical knowledge is scarce: An example of the use of partial least squares. In J. Kmenta and J. Ramsey (Eds.), *Evaluation of econometric models*. New York: Seminar, 1979.

Yaukey, D., Griffiths, W., and Roberts, B. J. Couple concurrence and empathy on birth control motivation in Dacca, East Pakistan. *American Sociological Review*, 1967, 32(5), 716-726.

4

The Second-Class Partner

THE MALE ROLE IN FAMILY-PLANNING DECISIONS

Raye Hudson Rosen and Twylah Benson

In the last few years, students of family planning have become increasingly aware of the "invisible man" and the possible significance of his part in fertility decision-making. With some notable exceptions, however, the bulk of fertility research has tended to focus on the female. Scholars who have been interested in the male role in family-planning decisions usually accepted the female partner's perceptions of that role, although we know that women's reports about their partners often do not jibe with reports from the men themselves (Heer, 1962; Kenkel, 1957; Nathanson, 1977; Safilios-Rothschild, 1969). The purpose of this chapter is to examine what information we have about the nature and extent of male participation in family-planning decisions in order to determine both how adequately we have been measuring that role and the extent to which the male needs to be a focus of research. One factor of paramount importance in making such an assessment is an analysis of the reasons that the male role frequently has been ignored.

In reviewing research that has dealt with the male role in family-planning decision-making, we shall divide the decisions into three major categories: (1) parenting decisions of married couples, which include whether and when to have children and how many to have; (2) decisions on contraceptive usage; and (3) decisions on resolution of pregnancies. There is, of course, overlap between parenting decisions and contraceptive decisions, but the studies that most logically can be included in the former category are broader than those focusing simply on whether or not birth control should be used.

PARENTING DECISIONS

Early Studies: Pre-1970

Much of the early family-planning research dealt with family size intentions of married couples, and, as such, sometimes used couples as research subjects (Kiser and Whelpton, 1953). A more common pattern was to contact only a portion of the husbands (Hill et al., 1959; Westoff et al., 1961). Most frequently, however, only wives were subjects, and their descriptions of their husbands' roles were accepted at face value. This was done even by some researchers who had found low correlations between husband and wife responses in some of their other studies (Stycos, 1968).

In terms of approach and findings of these studies, several points stand out. These studies typically did not consider the decision-making process per se. Most of the research that included husbands as respondents found discrepancies in the reports of husbands and wives (Bogue, 1962; Hill et al., 1959; Poti et al., 1962; Westoff et al., 1961). This seemed to have been the case in part because of lack of communication between spouses on subjects such as desired family size or wishes concerning contraception. In almost all cases where subjects were asked whether they had discussed such topics with their spouses, at least a third indicated no such conversations (Hill et al., 1959; Westoff et al., 1961). Often the proportion was much higher. For instance, in surveys conducted during 1963-1964 in various Latin American cities, nearly two-thirds of the female respondents in Bogotá and Caracas said they had never discussed ideal family size with their husbands (Stycos, 1971).

One of the consequences of such lack of communication was that wives often thought their husbands wanted more children than was the case. In several studies husbands were found to want as small, if not smaller, families as did their wives (Hill et al., 1959; Stycos, 1962).

Some researchers analyzed the bases for such lack of cummunication. Hill et al., (1959) concluded, for instance, that two barriers were critical in Puerto Rico: Wives' respect for husbands prevented discussion of intimate matters, and husbands believed that their wives were too modest to talk about such matters, although this was not really the case. Bogue (1962) indicated that many Indian husbands incorrectly perceived that their wives would not favor family planning, although they, themselves, were favorably disposed. The reasons that couples did not communicate with each other were comparable to those found in Puerto Rico. Mitchell (1972), in his large 1967 Hong Kong study, found that when there was disagreement between spouses on whether or not to have more children, the husband's opinion tended to prevail. A French survey (Michel, 1967) found that the more often the spouses discussed their problems, the more often they realized their family-planning goals. Communication was more important than socioeconomic variables in family-planning success, and this success was particularly associated with egalitarian or wife-dominant relations of the couples. Rainwater (1965) found discussion of family planning least common among lower-class blacks and most frequent among middle-class Protestants, in part because of their differing degrees of faith in the utility of contraception. Another factor in lack of communication was the husband's desire to make such decisions unilaterally. For example, in Puerto Rico, Hill et al. (1959) suggested that husbands often were afraid to allow their wives to take part in control of contraception because that might give them freedom to have sexual relations with other men.

Certainly, these studies indicated that men both desired and had an active role in family-planning decision-making. Perhaps this role should be seen within the context that the most commonly used birth-control methods of the time were male-based. Kirk pointed out in 1959 that the predominant use of methods requiring male initiative clearly did not suggest a lack of interest or willingness on the part of men to assume responsibility in this area (Kirk, 1959). Because of male dominance in such decision-making, a number of scholars suggested that family-planning education be directed primarily toward men (Bogue, 1962; Stycos, 1962, 1968).

Recent Studies: From 1970 On

While the focus of attention with respect to parenting decisions continues to be married couples, interest has expanded beyond studies of family size desires to include two new areas: the decision to remain voluntarily childless and how parenting decisions are affected by the perceived rewards and costs of children. Cross-nationally, however, studies of family size preference continue to be done as well. Although still not typical, a number of these have included the husband as a subject (Fisek and Sumbuloglu, 1978; Griffith, 1973; Nair and Chow, 1980; Scanzoni, 1975; Srinivasan et al., 1978).

Most of the earlier research on parenting decisions tended to presuppose a desire for children. In spite of a few exceptions (Centers and Blumberg, 1954; Kiser, 1939; Popenoe, 1936; Whelpton and Kiser, 1948), the vast bulk of research on voluntary childlessness has been done since 1970, and has continued to study parenting decisions only among married couples. Again, much of that research has involved only wives, who reported on themselves and their husbands (Houseknecht, 1977; Veevers, 1973; Welds, 1976). Even when both husbands and wives have been subjects, samples have tended to be unrepresentative and to lack control groups (Bram, 1978; Cooper et al., 1978; Marciano, 1979; Ory, 1978; Silka and Kiesler, 1977). Also, much of this research has concentrated on correlates of voluntary childlessness rather than on decision dynamics (Andrews and Withey, 1976; Barnett and MacDonald, 1976; Bram, 1978; Campbell et al., 1976; Gustavus and Henley, 1971; Magarick, 1976; Mai et al., 1972; Marcks, 1976; Nason and Poloma, 1976; Ory, 1978; Renne, 1976; Ritchey and Stokes, 1974; Veenhoven, 1974). One correlate particularly relevant to decision-making is that childless couples, compared to parents, have been found to have relatively egalitarian interactions with each other (Bram, 1978; Cooper et al., 1978; Veevers, 1975).

In spite of the methodological shortcomings noted above, a number of the voluntary childlessness studies have been suggestive with regard to the couples' decision dynamics. About a third of childless couples made the decision not to have children before marriage and, in effect, included a "childlessness clause" into their marriage contract (Veevers, 1973). Whether men or women, the individuals made their decisions without influence from a spouse. Cooper et al, (1978) found that about half of the couples who made a series of postponements of childbearing could be called "mutuals." That is, both partners came to the conclusion that childbearing was not for them at about the same time. They found among the remaining couples that one could distinguish between those in which the wife was more influential and those in which the husband had the greatest impact. Marciano (1979), on the other hand, suggested on the basis of several studies that, when the couples were not "mutuals," the husband tended either to have his way or to get a divorce. In very few cases of disagreement did the wife's desires prevail. This was found both for childless couples and for parents.

Another recent focus of parenting research has been on an examination of the perceived value of children, with a focus on social-psychological factors. To some extent, the expectancy or exchange theory approach used in recent work overlaps with the research on voluntary childlessness (Bram, 1978; Hamilton, 1976; Townes et al., 1976). Although males usually were included as subjects in this type of research, the common practice of sampling fewer males than females was followed in some of the major studies (Hoffman et al., 1978; Miller, 1980).

Both the perceived benefits and costs of having children often have been found to be similar for husbands and wives. Townes et al, (1976) found, however, that enhancing relations with relatives was a more significant value for wives than the experience of parenthood itself, while the reverse was true for husbands. Also, Tobin et al, (1975) found that the male view toward children coincided with both family size desires and with actual fertility more than was so for females. The authors (1975: 53) concluded that "it might logically be argued that a couple's fertility pattern is determined more by the husband's orientation toward children than by the wife's values."

CONTRACEPTIVE DECISIONS

Early Studies: Pre-1970

Many of the studies of married couples discussed in connection with parenting decisions also examined contraceptive decision-making (Hill and Back, 1959; Rainwater, 1960, 1965; Westoff et al., 1961). As noted, many of these studies gathered information only from wives (Freedman et al., 1959; Stycos, 1968; Whelpton et al., 1966) or, when husbands were included as subjects, sampled a smaller number of them than of wives (Bauman and Udry, 1972; Hill et al., 1959; Westoff et al., 1961). Quite a few of them examined husband-wife communication as a factor in effective contraception (Blake et al., 1969; Otero, 1968; Poffenberger and Poffenberger, 1973; Rainwater, 1960, 1965; Stycos, 1955), and found it to be significant.

Other studies were more narrowly focused on birth control per se, however. A number of these, particularly those done in developing countries, were interested in male attitudes and practices (Ahmed and Ahmed, 1965; Dandekar, 1963; Hong and Yoon, 1962; Morrison, 1957; Otero, 1968). Most of these studies focused on both male and female attitudes toward family planning, but a few dealt directly with decision-making. Otero (1968), for instance, in a national sample of 2,500 Mexican couples, found that rural-urban residence was related to type of decision-making on family planning. Unilateral male decisions were more typical among rural couples.

Among the more narrowly focused studies of birth control, those done in the United States rarely included males. Several studies of black males were notable exceptions to this pattern. Misra (1967) found that three quarters of the 118 low-income males studied approved of family planning, with those who were shy about sex less likely to approve of, be informed about, or practice contraception. In 1966, Bauman and Udry (1972) interviewed a sample of 350 married recent fathers and found a relatively strong negative relation between powerlessness and contraceptive regularity, even when other variables were controlled.

Recent Studies: 1970 On

Much recent research on contraceptive decision-making among married couples has continued to consider husband-wife communication about family planning and generally has supported the earlier findings of Hill et al. (1959) and Rainwater (1960, 1965) that such communication is positively associated with contraceptive use. As earlier, however, many of these studies had only female respondents and used their reports about communication between spouses (Kar and Talbot, 1980; Mukherjee, 1975; Phillips, 1978; World Health Organization Task Force, 1980). One methodologically and conceptually sophisticated study was done by Koenig (1980) in India. He wanted to determine the extent to which husband-wife communication was a casual factor in contraceptive use and the extent to which it was a mediating variable. It typically has been correlated with such variables as education, socioeconomic status, and modernity, all of which also are positively correlated with contraceptive use. Interviews were held with 1,598 couples in rural India in 1972. Koenig's major finding was that conjugal communication had little explanatory power of its own. He also discovered frequent differences between spouses as to whether communication about family planning had taken place, and that the probability of contraceptive use was markedly higher when spouses agreed that they had discussed the subject. Such communication generally took the form of directives from the husband to his wife. Another methodologically sophisticated study of fertility decision-making, which included decision-making on birth control, was done by Beckman (1980) with a sample of 578 husbands and an equal number of wives. Reports of spouses as to who made decisions regarding birth control differed significantly from one another, as did their beliefs about which spouse should make such decisions. Husbands tended to indicate that both spouses should and did take responsibility for preventing unwanted pregnancies; wives, on the other hand, reported that they alone had that responsibility, but agreed that it *should* be a mutual one.

During the last decade many studies of contraceptive decisions also have begun to deal with unmarried individuals and quite a few, although still a minority, have included males in the samples. When single males have been subjects, samples typically have been of college populations and males have been sampled equally with females. These males have not been partners of the female subjects, however. Also, most have been convenience samples (Cole and Allen, 1979; Delamater and MacCorquodale, 1978; Fox and Fox, 1976; Kelley, 1979; Thompson and Spanier, 1978). A number of them have focused on personality variables as possible predictors of birth-control usage. For instance, Miller (1980) used five scales and found that they predicted contraceptive behavior better for males than for females, especially the risk-taking scale. This agrees with the findings of Cvetkovich et al. (1975) in their investigations of high school students, except that they found that both males and females who were poor contraceptive users were oriented toward risk-taking. Both sex role orientation and focus of control have been variables of interest as well. Fox (1977) found that neither predicted contraceptive behavior of male university student respondents, although both, in conjunction with each other, did predict for females. In another study, Fox and Fox (1976) found that males were more likely to contracept with feminine than with androgynous women. Delamater and Mac-Corquodale (1978) also found differences in predictors of contraceptive use for males and females. They tried to test two models — Rain's (1971) model of moral ambivalence and Reiss's (1967) model of acceptance of one's own sexuality — and found neither applicable to male contraceptive activity. Thompson and Spanier (1978) looked at the relative influence of parents, peers, and partners on contraceptive use and found that partner influence was predominant for males, while the pattern for females was more complex. Weinstein and Goebel (1979), like Cole and Allen (1979), hypothesized that men who were more positive toward male contraception would subscribe less strongly to stereotypic beliefs that birth control was a woman's responsibility. Their hypothesis was supported with data from a non-random sample. In addition, they found that married and more educated men tended to have more positive attitudes toward male birth control than others. Many of these studies examined communication between partners as perceived by one partner as a variable in contraceptive use, and they generally agreed with earlier studies of married couples that there was a positive relationship between the two variables (Cole and Allen, 1979; Delamater and MacCorquodale, 1978; Fox, 1976). Stable, continuing relationships also were found to be a major predictor of contraceptive use (Cvetkovich and Grote, 1976, 1977; Delamater and MacCorquodale, 1978; Foreit and Foreit, 1978; Furstenberg, 1976; Sterns and Garland, 1979).

When we look at studies of contraceptive decisions among minors, we again find that few have included male partners, although male methods account for nearly half of teenage contraception (Scales, 1977). Research on such males typically has described their attitudes and behavior (Arnold, 1972; Finkel and Finkel, 1975; Gilbert and Matthews, 1974; Miller, 1973; Ross, 1979). Usually, however, researchers concerned with contraceptive practices and/or decisions of adolescents have followed the traditional practice of using the female's report on her relationship with her male partner(s) and how this may have affected her decision to use birth control (Bracken et al., 1978a, 1978b; Ewer and Gibbs, 1975; Furstenberg, 1976; Jorgensen et al., 1980; Lindeman, 1974; Zelnick and Kantner, 1977). Generally, they have found that the closer and more stable the female reports the relationship to be, the more likely she is to have used contraceptives. The only studies to date which have used adolescent couples are those of the authors (Benson, 1981), Meara (1980), and Polit (1980).

Benson (1981) examined 33 couples and found that 58 percent (18) of the dyads had used birth control before the pregnancy occurred, and that all of these dyads agreed on the method used. Sometimes one member of a dyad mentioned using more methods than his or her partner. Almost a quarter (23 percent) used condoms only, and half used condoms and something else. Also, almost half of the dyads agreed that both partners should be responsible for contraception, while about a third (34 percent) disagreed over whose responsibility it should be. Benson had hypothesized that males' traditional sex role attitudes would be positively associated with a belief that the female should be responsible for contraception. The hypothesis was not supported. In addition, no differences in beliefs about contraceptive responsibility were found for those who chose abortion as a pregnancy resolution choice, compared to those who chose to have the child kept. These findings agree with other research with respect to discrepancies between partners in norms for contraceptive responsibility (Beckman, 1980), and reinforce the conclusion that males have an important role in the contraceptive decision.

PREGNANCY RESOLUTION DECISIONS

Early Studies: Pre-1970

Since elective abortion was not legal anywhere in the United States prior to 1970, most early studies of pregnancy resolution dealt with keeping the child versus releasing it for adoption. These studies dealt entirely with unmarried individuals, and rarely either included the male partner as a subject or even considered the female's perception of his part in the decision-making (Bowerman et al., 1966; Rains, 1971; Vincent, 1961). One of the few studies that recognized abortion as a pregnancy resolution alternative was Nancy Lee's (1969) research on illegal abortions. She had to use enormous ingenuity to find appropriate female subjects. Consequently, she made no effort to include male partners, but did report on the female perceptions of the male role and her relationship with her partner. The few early studies in which the male partner was an object of research tended to focus only on situations where the child was borne and to use convenience samples. For instance, Pannor et al. (1971) obtained data during the early 1960s from partners of unmarried mothers who were receiving counseling at a Jewish agency for children. Platt's (1968) subjects were partners of single mothers seeking adoption services. In such studies, contact with the male generally was made through the female. If she had lost contact with him or did not wish him to be involved, the investigators had no means of access to him.

Recent Studies: 1970 On

Although interest in pregnancy resolution decision-making has burgeoned since 1970, studies have concentrated on unmarried populations and have rarely included males in their samples. Failure to use male subjects has generally not been due to lack of awareness of the importance of the male role in such decision-making, however. Rather, it has resulted from the difficulties of reaching male partners of single women, especially those who either do not know about the pregnancy or who do not care to be involved in the resolution of it. In cases where the pregnancy has precipitated a break in the relationship, female respondents often do not wish to have the relevant male contacted. Consequently, many researchers have tended to obtain information about the pregnant female's perceptions of her relationship with the man involved and how this affected her decision-making, as well as, in some cases, data on his perceived part in the decision-making (Blumenfield, 1978; Bracken et al., 1978a, 1978b; Cobliner et al., 1973; Evans and Nathanson, 1977; Fischman, 1977; McCormick, 1975; Monsour and Stewart, 1973; Pearson, 1973; Perez-Reyes and Falk, 1973; Rosen, 1976; Schaffer and Pine, 1972).

The few studies that included males have predominantly used the partners of aborters (Peled, 1978; Rothstein, 1977; Shostak, 1979). No studies except that of Peled (1978) and that of the authors have been found which used couples as the unit of analysis. Although Rothstein (1977) was interested in understanding the relationships of couples seeking abortion, the men and women studied were not selected as couples.

Let us turn to what has been found, both from women's reports and the studies that examined males directly. Most studies found that pregnant women tended to tell their partners about their pregnancies (Chandler, 1975; MacIntrye, 1977; McCormick, 1975; Pearson, 1973; Perez-Reyes and Falk, 1973; Rosen, 1976; Zimmerman, 1977). They also typically found that the nature of the dyad's relationship was a critical factor in the decision-making. For instance, women who delivered and kept the child generally were found to have longer and/or more stable relationships with their male partners than was the case for aborters (Bracken et al., 1978b; Fischman, 1977; Pearson, 1973; Robbins, 1980). On the other hand, a number of researchers have reported that their subjects decided to get an abortion either because of an unstable relationship with a man or because of a threat to the relationship if the child were kept (Browner, 1975; Cobliner et al., 1973; Fischman, 1977; McCormick, 1975; Monsour and Stewart, 1973; Pearson, 1973; Steinhoff, 1978). Zimmerman (1977) pointed out that male partners in such relationships were influential in the decision, but only in a negative way, by closing off the alternative of marriage or a continuing relationship if the child was kept. Others have indicated another way in which the male in an unstable relationship was negatively influential: Because the woman did not want to marry her partner or have his child, she chose abortion (Shaw et al., 1979; Steinhoff, 1978). There are almost no systematic data on the nature of the relationship and its stability among those few who decided to bear a child and release it for adoption.

One cannot necessarily extrapolate from the nature of the relationship to the extent of active male involvement in the decision-making, however. There is no consensus in what has been found. Some researchers have concluded that women tend to exclude men from their decision-making, making their choices independently, even though male partners may have been used as a source of support (Fischman, 1977; Schaffer and Pine, 1972; Zimmerman, 1977). Others have indicated that male partners may have been involved in the decision-making but often were not supportive (Bogen, 1974; McCormick, 1975; Shaw et al., 1979). Some found that women who delivered were more likely to have involved their partner than did women who aborted, as well as more likely to receive support from him (Bracken et al., 1978b; Fischman, 1977), while others reported mutual decision-making and agreement on a solution from most couples whose final choice was abortion (Peled, 1978; Shostak, 1979; Steinhoff, 1978). Still others found the impact of partners applied to part of the group studied, often about half (Rosen, 1976; Rothstein, 1977).

Many researchers have tended to assume that partner support would be a valuable aid to the pregnant woman. Several others have questioned that, however. For instance, Kerman (1975) pointed out that involvement of the man in the decision-making often led to early marriage and to another early pregnancy, and there is considerable evidence that early marriage and childbearing have a number of negative consequences, including early divorce (Arnold and Hoffman, 1974; Brunswick, 1971; Furstenberg, 1976; Trussell, 1976). Chandler (1975) found that the participation and support of the male partner, as well as his presence at the abortion clinic, were positively associated with anxiety of the woman at the time of abortion. Women who went to the abortion clinic alone reported the least anxiety. She suggested that perhaps those who were least anxious could best afford to go through the procedure alone. She also concluded, however, that it "seemed as if the more the decision was initiated by women, left up to them, and favored by them, the less anxious they were. . . . Perhaps because women are so often delegated full responsibility for pregnancies, etc. they do not benefit from support very much. Instead, they feel as if it is their problem alone, no matter who is there for them" (1975: 92).

ROSEN-BENSON DATA ON MALE PARTNERS OF ADOLESCENTS[1]

In our own research among adolescents, we have examined the male role in pregnancy resolution decision-making both from the perspective of the female and from that of her partner. The population studied was a rural one, with primarily white subjects, as was representative of the area. The female respondents were patients of private physicians, the only medical care givers within the county. Since the county did not have medical clinics, the study population consisted of all pregnant teenagers who were served within the county during a 14-month period and their partners.

As has been noted for other research, a major problem in the fieldwork was gaining access to and cooperation from males. There were 100 female respondents, but it was possible to reach only 33 of the male partners. Of those, 19 were interviewed. The remainder completed a structured questionnaire covering most of the same items as the interview. In contrast to some of the studies noted earlier, however, the smaller number of males was not intended. In 27 cases the female did not want her partner contacted, and in 16 cases the males refused to participate. The remaining 24 partners could not be reached for various reasons, ranging from having moved away from the area to loss of contact with the female before she had asked her partner to cooperate.

Let us look first at the female's perception of her partner's role in the decision-making. The female subjects included 64 who had decided to abort and 31 who had decided to keep the child.[2] Of the male respondents, two-thirds were partners of aborters, while the other third were partners of women who planned to keep their babies.

We categorized the impact of the male partner upon the pregnancy resolution decision-making in four ways: direct pressure, indirect pressure, direct influence, and indirect influence. By direct pressure we meant the explicit use of resources as a potential or actual weapon in order to gain compliance with what is desired. For the male partner, this tended to be threats of breaking off the relationship or withholding financial help, as well as refusal of marriage when the female partner wanted that option, and suasion by dominance of manner *toward* marriage which the female partner originally did not want. Indirect pressure referred to the subject's fear that resources might be used as a weapon, and her consequent behavior in terms of avoiding such an outcome. Direct influence meant advice given with a promise of support regardless of the outcome chosen. It included the male partner's willingness to facilitate all options, including marriage. By indirect influence we meant situational factors not directly associated with the decision-making but providing a limitation or a perspective within which the subject decided. Such situational factors in the case of male partners included (1) circumstances that prevented the option of marriage, such as his being married, the pregnancy resulting from a "one-night stand," the couple having broken up, the female's lack of interest in marrying him, their mutual lack of interest in marrying; (2) circumstances that led to a perspective that there was no decision to be made (that is, it was taken for granted the child would be kept); for many respondents and their partners, although not all, being married or engaged meant that one never even questioned keeping the child; (3) the respondent's concern for her partner's welfare, as she saw it, without any input concerning it from him; she felt he could not afford a child, was too young to marry, and so on, and made her decision independently, but with such considerations as a major element in what she chose. The latter category could be considered as consisting of males who were not involved at all in the decision-making. They, and the few in the indirect pressure cateogry, were not active participants in the solving of a problem. Since situations relating to them or to their relationship with the respondents affected the decision that was made, however, it seemed more useful to explore how those situations may have been important than to dismiss these males as uninvolved.

The most common form of impact female subjects perceived their partners to have on their pregnancy resolution decision was *indirect influence,* with 41 percent falling in that category. Indirect influence was more common among partners of women who kept their children (52 percent) than among partners of women who aborted (34 percent).

The perspective that there was no problem and no decision to be made was the most important form of indirect influence among couples who kept the child. Although the pregnancy was not planned, no alternatives to keeping the child usually were considered, either for those married before the pregnancy occured or for those who planned to marry later. Circumstances that prevented marriage were the predominant indirect influence for partners of aborters (87 percent).

Direct Influence characterized 29 percent of the male partners: one-third (34 percent) of aborters' partners and close to one-fifth (19 percent) of partners of women who kept the child. The most frequent form of direct influence found (among 71 percent of the keepers, and 67 percent of the aborters) was for couples to explore alternatives together, as illustrated in the following example. A 19-year-old who chose abortion described the couple's decision-making process: "Since we talked about it, we both came up with the same answers and the same feelings about it." The remaining one-third of the male partners who directly influenced the decision deferred to the female's choice, after offering their own opinions. This is illustrated by a 16-year-old who kept the baby. She reported: "He feels like he wished it didn't happen right now, but he said he'll go along with anything I want to do. It's my life."

Of the female respondents, 27 percent indicated *direct pressure* on their pregnancy resolution decision from their male partners. They were fairly evenly split between those who aborted and those who kept the child. The pregnancy outcome groups differed in the proportions of males who were successful in their pressure. Only one-third of the pressuring partners of women who kept the child were totally successful. (The remainder included four who urged abortion and two who wanted marriage as well as the child being kept.) Two-thirds were successful with aborters. Their success in persuading their partners to abort rested mainly on the females' desire to maintain the relationship. *All* who acceded to direct pressure to abort would have preferred to marry and keep the child if their partner had been willing. On the other hand, with one exception, the partners of aborters who were unsuccessful in applying direct pressure urged marriage and keeping the child. The one exception wanted his partner to release the child for adoption rather than have an abortion.

Only 3 percent of the male partners exerted *indirect pressure*. This was a proportion too small for any meaningful analysis.

Turning to the male respondents' report of their role in the decision-making,[3] it is important to note at the outset that 77 percent of the males who were willing to cooperate in the study were perceived by their partners to have actively participated in the decision-making process. This means that, although they were a small subset of the male partners, they were an important group to examine with respect to their role in the pregnancy resolution choice. By and large, they were a significant factor in the couple's decision-making, and this was not true for many of the male nonrespondents.

Some of the studies that included males have suggested that about 40 percent of sexually active males had never even considered the possibility that their female partners might become pregnant (Schofield, 1965; Sorenson, 1973). The same pattern held for our respondents, and even those who had thought about the possibility had not developed any real contingency plans for such an eventuality.

The number and type of pregnancy resolution alternatives that male partners considered were also examined. Only 22 percent did not think of any alternatives to their final choices, and 29 percent considered at least four alternatives. It was interesting to find that 80 percent of those who were married or engaged considered alternatives to keeping the child, rather than simply taking such a position for granted. The alternative most commonly considered by all male respondents was abortion (90 percent); getting married and keeping the child were second (84 percent). When thinking about abortion, respondents tended to see more rewards than costs, but thought about both cost and rewards more often than was the case with other alternatives. Those who wanted their partner to have an abortion saw both more rewards and more costs for this action than did those who wanted their partner to keep the child. When keeping the child was considered, however, those who wanted their partner to take this action saw mostly rewards of doing so, while those who desired abortion saw more costs of keeping the child. The most important benefit of abortion, as they saw it, was being able to keep the pregnancy secret, while second in importance was avoiding the financial burden of childbearing and rearing. The major cost of abortion was perceived to be trauma for the female partner. When marriage and keeping the child were considered, the major reward mentioned was the opportunity to be together as a committed pair, and the second reward, mentioned almost as often, was the pleasure of having a child. The most common cost was perceived to be having to get married. Second came both interruption of future plans and not being ready for the responsibility involved. The most important reward of staying single but having the partner keep the child was seen as having the pleasure of a child. The most frequently mentioned cost was the difficulty the female would have in raising a child alone. None expressed a desire to raise the child himself. Only 12 respondents thought about adoption as an alternative, but for those who did, the two rewards cited most often were avoiding marriage and avoiding the responsibilities of parenthood. Respondents saw almost four times as many costs as rewards for this alternative, however, and the most frequently mentioned cost was loss of the child.

Next we looked at several factors associated with the male partner's decision on how the pregnancy should be resolved. Choice of abortion was positively related to high educational goals and social class, desire to keep the pregnancy secret, and definition of the pregnancy as a crisis. These factors were related to each other as well; aborters with high educational goals tended to come from middle-class backgrounds and to perceive the pregnancy as a crisis. Catholicism also was positively related to choice of abortion.

Turning to the impact of significant others on the male's choice of pregnancy resolution, we found the major form of *parental* impact to be *indirect pressure,* primarily in the form of feared disapproval. *Direct influence* was next in importance, mainly in the form of parents' discussion of the various alternatives with their son, with assurances of support regardless of the son's choice. Some *indirect influence* from parents was reported and took two forms. One was an atmosphere of acceptance of the pregnancy, with joy about becoming grandparents. The other was the respondents' memory of parents' reactions to earlier teenage pregnancies of their sibling. Finally, a number of male partners indicated *direct pressure* from parents. Most of this pressure was toward abortion, as has been reported in the literature for females. These parents were concerned about their child's future. A fifth of the males reported that parents had *no influence* on their decision.

The major form of impact by *sibs* was *indirect influence* through their involvement in one or more pregnancies. Forty-eight percent of the male respondents reported that at least one sibling had been involved in a minor's pregnancy. Although only about one-half of such males made the same choice as their sibs had made, there was some evidence that unsuccessful resolution of a sibling pregnancy influenced the male to make a different decision. There was also some *direct influence* on the decision by siblings. In most of these cases a sister who previously had been involved in such a pregnancy discussed the various alternatives with the male and/or gave advice. *Indirect influence* also was the major form of impact by *peers,* but *direct influence* ran a close second.

The most important source of impact, as might be expected, was the *female partner.* The great majority of males (82 percent) described the female partner's effect on their choice as one of *direct influence.* Most of them indicated that they had talked the problem over and discussed the various alternatives. For example, "We talked about how it would be to be married — what it would be like and how it would affect our relationship when we're so young. And we talked about how much easier it would be to have an abortion instead of getting married." Some had discussed possible alternatives before the female partner even became pregnant. As one reported, "We talked about it a long time ago — that if she did get pregnant she'd have an abortion — as far as parents were concerned and school." In a few cases, the young woman simply told her partner what she wanted to do and he was accepting of her wish. For each of the other three categories, only one respondent reported that type of impact.

Finally, the impact of the male partner on the female was examined from the male perspective and compared to the perspective of his partner (presented earlier). Eighty-eight percent of the male respondents viewed their impact on the female as direct influence. Most of them reported discussing the alternatives either before or after she became pregnant, and reaching an agreement on the decision. Only two respondents reported their impact as indirect influence. In one such case there simply was an assumption that they would keep the child and that no decision had to be made. He exclaimed, "We planned on getting married anyway, before she got pregnant. I definitely planned on keeping the child. I was proud of it." When data from the female interviews for those whose partners were respondents were compared to the data from the male interviews, considerable differences were found. While none of the males described their impact as of the more threatening types, direct pressure or indirect pressure, 47 percent of the females saw their partners as using these forms of suasion. Also, about a third (35 percent) of the females saw their partners' impact as direct influence. In other words, the females generally saw the males' impact as more forceful than the males themselves did. A Wilcoxon matched-pairs signed ranks test indicated that these differences were significant. Of the males who were perceived by their female partners as exerting direct pressure, 80 percent were reported to be successful in their outcome. Most of them (60 percent) pressured the female to abort and she did so. All of that pressure was in terms of a threat to break off the relationship if the female partner did not comply with the male's wishes. A bargain was struck, with maintenance of the relationship the female's reward in return for the cost of aborting the pregnancy. Both the differing perceptions of partners and the dominance of male desires in case of disagreement agreed with many other studies that have been discussed in this chapter.

SUMMARY AND CONCLUSIONS

It appears that there have been and continue to be many methodological shortcomings in studying the male role in family-planning decisions, but that these have varied considerably among the differing types of decisions.

There seems to be no intrinsic reasons that male cooperation equal to that of female cannot be obtained in parenting decisions, at least among the married, which is the primary group that has been studied. The fact that female reports of the male role in parenting decisions have tended to be used, or that fewer male than female subjects have been sampled in such research, does not seem to have occurred as the result of insuperable barriers to obtaining married male respondents. Rather, it seems to indicate that many researchers have operated in terms of cultural biases, assuming that the male's role is less important in parenting decisions than that of the female. Since the findings from a number of studies where the male was included in some way reveal considerable discrepancies between men's and women's reports of the same event, as well as male dominance in most decision-making, it seems rather odd that researchers have continued to downplay the male's role. If parenting decisions were studied among single people, it might be more difficult to obtain both individuals in a dyad than would be the case with married couples. We cannot be sure of this, however, unless and until such needed research is initiated.

With respect to contraceptive decision-making, the bulk of studies have concentrated on women, even prior to the development of the Pill and the interuterine device. What evidence we have of the male role in contraceptive decisions is equivocal, with some studies indicating active male interest in birth-control decisions, especially within a stable relationship with communication, and others indicating considerable disinterest, particularly among the young and less educated. Lack of male interest may be a predominant factor in noncontraception, however, and needs to be studied as much as does active concern. Quite a few studies of contraception using single people as subjects have examined such dimensions, but generally not for couples per se. The report of either the man or the woman regarding such relevant variables as the nature of the couple relationship has tended to be taken at face value. Considerably more comparison of couples' perspectives needs to be made. The difficulties of obtaining cooperation from single and/or adolescent couples may be considerably greater than with adult spouses, but this cannot really be determined until some attempts at such research have been made.

In recent years, studies of pregnancy resolution decisions have tended to recognize the importance of the male role in the decision-making, but, because of barriers to obtaining his cooperation, have tended to use the female's perception of his role. When studying the pregnancy resolution decision, it is almost impossible to avoid recognition of the importance of using couples, but the need to use males who are partners of pregnant respondents is the source of a major difficulty in obtaining male subjects. One cannot logically use a randomly selected population, as frequently may be done in studies of desired family size, value of children, and contraceptive decisions. Individuals who have not been involved in a pregnancy cannot answer meaningfully about what their role in resolution decisions might be. Consequently, as is the case with the decision to remain voluntarily childless, the population of interest is a very restricted, specialized one, difficult to locate and obtain cooperation from. Obviously, it is easier to find female than male subjects, since pregnant women tend to go to predictable caregivers for assistance. Some researchers have studied males who accompanied their female partners to such caregivers — particularly those waiting in abortion clinics. Such men are a minor proportion of the partners of aborters, however. Most researchers who have attempted to obtain males as subjects have sought access to them through their female partners. There are various problems with this approach: the female may not have told the male about her pregnancy; she may not wish the male to be contacted even if he knows about the pregnancy; he may not wish to be contacted due to indifference or fear of the consequences. As a result, most who are secured in that way are a sample biased in favor of those most actively involved in the decision process. One should not despair, however; this is an important group to study and researchers might profitably settle for contact with such males as a first step. One group that might be of particular interest to approach is husbands in states that require spousal consent for abortion (Karg, 1978).

In trying to assess the reasons that the male role frequently has been downplayed, a major factor seems to have been a general lack of concern with decision dynamics, which frequently would involve couples. The fact that it is the woman who gets pregnant and must deal with that pregnancy also seems to have led to the assumption that family planning is less salient to the male than to his partner. This seems to spring in part from the use of a medical model re contraception, pregnancy, and maternal health. Such a model traditionally has focused on the individual patient. It is reinforced by the advent of such female-based contraceptives as the Pill and the interuterine device, and the perspective by family-planning specialists that these are the most effective devices. In addition, however, it would appear that researchers' unconscious acceptance of sex role stereotypes is a factor. Family and children are assumed to be the domain of women, with first priority for them, but of secondary concern to men. Unconscious bias also appears to have been operating when researchers have ignored both single males and females in studies of parenting decisions, although there is evidence from other types of research that parenthood may be valued and sought among certain groups of single people (Furstenberg, n.d.; Sabe and Wikler, 1979; Stack, 1974).

Not only is there a need to include the male in all studies of family-planning decision-making, and to focus more on the process of such decision-making, but it is important to use couples as a unit of analysis. It may be worthwhile to point out some of the methodological problems of doing so, however. Not only is access to the male difficult to obtain, but, once it is secured, the resulting differences in responses must be dealt with. Which partner's report can be presumed to be more reliable for variables such as degree of communication or degree and nature of influence on a family-planning decision? Are the differences in perception examined without regard to the issue of reliability? In other cases, of course, such as family size desires, the differences in responses may simply indicate disagreement between the partners.

There have been a number of indications in recent years that researchers in the area of family planning have been increasingly concerned about including the male directly in their studies (American Public Health Association, 1980; Psychosocial Factors in Population Research, 1980). This is promising, if some of the methodological barriers to doing so effectively can be overcome.

NOTES

1. The research was supported by Grant HD-ll099, NICHD, and Grant 78-499, Stewart Mott Foundation.

2. Four who were undecided at the time of the first interview were not included in these analyses.

3. The analyses of male data were drawn from Twylah Benson's Ph. D. dissertation, *Impregnators of Teenagers and Their Part in the Pregnancy Resolution Decision,* Wayne State University, 1981. Data on males were collected under Grant 78-499, Stewart Mott Foundation.

REFERENCES

Ahmed, M., and Ahmed, F. Male attitudes toward family limitation in East Pakistan. *Eugenics Quarterly,* 1965, 12, 209-226.

American Public Health Association. Male involvement in the use of contraception. Program for the annual meeting of the APHA, Detroit, Michigan, October 21, 1980.

Andrews, F. J., and Withey, S. B. *Social indicators of well-being: Americans' perceptions of life quality.* New York: Plenum, 1976.

Arnold, C. B. The sexual behavior of inner city adolescent condom users. *Journal of Sex Research,* 1972, 8, 298-309.

Arnold, S., and Hoffman, A. Chicago planned parenthood's teen scene: A sociological study for participants. *Adolescence,* 1974, 9 (Fall), 371-390.

Barnett, L. D., and MacDonald, R. H. A study of the membership of the National Organization for Non-parents. *Social Biology,* 1976, 23 (Winter), 297-310.

Bauman, K. E., and Udry, J. R. Powerlessness and regularity of contraception in an urban negro male sample. A research note. *Journal of Marriage and the Family,* 1972, 34, 112-114.

Beckman, L. J. *The relative influence of husband versus wife in fertility decision-making.* Paper presented at the Eighth Annual Workshop on Psychosocial Factors in Population Research, April 8-9, Denver, Colorado, 1980.

Benson, T. Impregnators of teenagers and their part in the pregnancy resolution decision. Doctoral dissertation, Wayne State University, 1981.

Blake, R. R., Insko, C. A., Cialdini, R. B., and Chaikin, A. L. *Beliefs and attitudes about contraception among the poor.* Chapel Hill, NC: Carolina Population Center, 1969.

Blumenfield, M. Psychological factors involved in request for elective abortion. *Journal of Clinical Psychiatry,* 1978, 39, 17-25.

Bogen, I. Attitudes of women who have had abortions. *Journal of Sex Research,* 1974, 10, 97-109.

Bogue, D.J. Some tentative recommendations for a "sociologically correct" family planning communication and motivation program in India. In C. V. Kiser (Ed.), *Research in family planning.* Princeton, NJ: Princeton University Press, 1962.

Bowerman, C., Irish, D., and Pope, H. *Unwed motherhood: Personal and social consequences.* Chapel Hill, NC: Institute for Research in Social Science, University of North Carolina, 1966.

Bracken, M. B., Klerman, L. V., and Bracken, M. Abortion, adoption, or motherhood: An empirical study of decision-making during pregnancy. *American Journal of Obstetrics and Gynecology,* 1978, 130(3), 251-262.(a)

Bracken, M. B., Klerman, L. V., and Bracken, M. Coping with pregnancy resolution among never-married women. *American Journal of Orthopsychiatry,* 1978, 48(2), 320-334.(b)

Bram, S. Through the looking glass: Voluntary childlessness as a mirror for contemparary changes in the meaning of parenthood. In W. B. Miller and L. F. Newman (Eds.), *The first child and family formation.* Chapel Hill, NC: Carolina Population Center, 1978.

Browner, C. *Abortion as a life crisis.* 1975. (Mimeo; see *The Papers of the Kroeber Anthropological Society,* 1975, 47).

Brunswick, A. F. Adolescent health, sex and fertility: Adolescent sexuality and its problems, particularly pregnancy. *American Journal of Public Health,* 1971, 61(4), 711-729.

Campbell, A., Converse, P.E., and Rodgers, W.L. *The quality of American life: Perceptions, evaluations, and satisfactions.* New York: Russell Sage, 1976.

Centers, R., and Blumberg, G. H. Social and psychological factors in human procreation. *Journal of Social Psychology,* 1954, 40(2), 245-257.

Chandler, L.J. Women's social networks: Their effects on the anxiety of abortion. Doctoral dissertation, University of Michigan, 1975.

Cobliner, W. G., Schulman, H., and Romney, S. L. The termination of adolescent out-of-wedlock pregnancies and the prospects for their primary prevention. *American Journal of Obstetrics and Gynecology,* 1973, 115(3), 432-444.

Cole, J. B., and Allen, F. C. L. Contraceptive responsibility among male university students. *Journal of the Australian College Health Association,* 1979, 28, 168-172.

Cooper, P.E., Cumber, B., and Hartner, R. Decision-making patterns and post decision adjustment of childfree husbands and wives. *Alternative Lifestyles,* 1978, 1 (February), 71-94.

Cvetkovich, G., and Grote, B. *Psychological factors associated with adolescent premarital coitus.* Paper presented at the National Institute of Child Health and Human Development, Bethesda, Maryland, 1976.

Cvetkovich, G., and Grote, B. *Adolescent development and teenage fertility.* Paper presented at the Planned Parenthood Regional Conference on Adolescence, Boise, Idaho, June 16,1977.

Cvetkovich, G., Grote, B., Bjorseth, A., and Sarkissian, J. On the psychology of adolescents' use of contraceptives. *Journal of Sex Research,* 1975, 11(3), 256-269.

Dandekar, K. Vasectomy camps in Maharashtra. *Population Studies,* 1963, 17, 147-154.

Delamater, J., and MacCorquodale, P. Premarital contraceptive use: A test of two models. *Journal of Marriage and the Family,* 1978, 40(2), 235-247.

Evans, A. R., and Nathanson, C. A. *Late abortion among teenagers.* Paper presented at the Annual Meeting of the American Public Health Association, Washington, D.C., October 31, 1977.

Ewer, P., and Gibbs, J. Relationship with father and use of contraception in a population of black ghetto adolescent mothers. *Public Health Reports,* 1975, 90 (September), 417-423.

Finkel, M. L., and Finkel, J. Sexual and contraceptive knowledge, attitudes and behavior of male adolescents. *Family Planning Perspectives,* 1975 7(6), 256-260.

Fischman, S. Delivery or abortion in inner-city adolescents. *American Journal of Orthopsychiatry,* 1977, 47(1), 127-133.

Fisek, N. H., and Sumbuloglu, K. The effects of husband and wife education on family planning in rural Turkey. *Studies in Family Planning,* 1978, 9(10-11), 280-285.

Foreit, K. G., and Foreit, J. R. Correlates of contraceptive behavior among unmarried U.S. college students. *Studies in Family Planning,* 1978, 9(6), 169-174.

Fox, B. R., and Fox, G. L. *The contraceptive and sexual behavior of feminine and androgynous women.* Paper presented at the annual meetings of the National Council on Family Relations, San Diego, 1976.

Fox, G. L. *Accounting for patterns of contraceptive use and nonuse among unmarried college students.* Detroit: Merrill-Palmer Institute.

Fox, G. L. Sex-role attitudes as predictors of contraceptive use among unmarried university students. *Sex Roles: A Journal of Research,* 1977, 3(3), 265-283.

Freedman, R., Whelpton, P. K., and Campbell, A. A. *Family planning, sterility and population growth.* New York: McGraw-Hill, 1959.

Furstenberg, F. F., Jr. *Unplanned parenthood.* New York: Free Press, 1976.

Furstenberg, F. F., Jr. *Children's names and paternal claims: Bonds between unmarried fathers and their children.* Philadelphia: University of Pennsylvania, n.d.

Gilbert, R., and Matthews, V. G. Young males' attitudes toward condom use. In M. A. Redford, G. W. Duncan, and D. J. Prager (Eds.), *The condom: Increasing utilization in the United States.* San Francisco: San Francisco Press, 1974.

Griffith, J. Social pressure on family size intentions. *Family Planning Perspectives,* 1973, 5(4), 237-242.

Gustavus, S. O., and Henley, J. R., Jr. Correlates of voluntary childlessness in a select population. *Social Biology,* 1971, 18 (September), 277-284.

Hamilton, M. R. Application of a utility-cost decision model to a comparison of intentionally childless couples and parent couples (Doctoral dissertation, University of Maryland, 1976). *Dissertation Abstracts,* 1976, 38, 2360A.

Heer, D. M. Husband and wife perceptions of family power structures. *Marriage and Family Living,* 1962, 24, 65-67.

Hill, R., Stycos, J. M., and Back, K. W. *The family and population control: A Puerto Rican experiment in social change.* Chapel Hill, NC: University of North Carolina Press, 1959.

Hoffman, L. W., Thornton, A., and Manis, J. D. The value of children to parents in the United States. *Journal of Population,* 1978, 1, 93-131.

Hong, S. B., and Yoon, J. H. Male attitudes toward family planning on the island of Kangwha-Gun, Korea. *Millbank Memorial Fund Quarterly,* 1962, 40, 443-452.

Houseknecht, S. H. Wives but not mothers: Factors influencing the decision to remain voluntarily childless (Doctoral dissertation, Pennsylvania State University, 1977). *Dissertation Abstracts,* 1977, 38, 6345A.

Jorgensen, S., King, S., and Torrey, B. Dyadic and social network influences on adolescent exposure to pregnancy risk. *Journal of Marriage and the Family,* 1980, 42(1), 141-155.

Kar, S. B., and Talbot, J. M. Attitudinal and nonattitudinal determinants of contraception: A cross-cultural study. *Studies in Family Planning,* 1980, 11 (2) 51-64.

Karg, B. Restrictions on women's right to abortion: Informed consent, spousal consent, and recordkeeping provisions. *Women's Rights Law Reporter,* 1978, 5(1), 35-51.

Kelley, K. Socialization factors in contraceptive attitudes: Roles of affective responses, parental attitudes and sexual experience. *Journal of Sex Research,* 1979, 15, 6-20.

Kenkel, W. F. Influence differentiation in family decision-making. *Sociology and Social Research,* 1957, 42, 18-25.

Kirk, D. *Possible lessons from historical experience for family planning programs in Asia.* Paper presented at the Sixth International Conference on Planned Parenthood, London, 1959.

Kiser, C. V. Voluntary and unvoluntary aspects of childlessness. *Millbank Memorial Fund Quarterly,* 1939, 17 (January), 50-68.

Kiser, C. V., and Whelpton, P. K. Resume of the Indianapolis study of social and psychological factors affecting fertility. *Population Studies,* 1953, 7, 95-110.

Klerman, L. V. Adolescent pregnancy: The need for new policies and new programs. *Journal of School Health,* 1975, 45(5), 263-267.

Koenig, M. A. *Husband-wife interaction and contraceptive adoption in rural India.* Paper presented at the Eighth Annual Workshop on Psycho-Social Factors in Population Research, April 8-9, Denver, Colorado, 1980.

Lee, N. *The search for an abortionist.* Chicago: University of Chicago Press, 1969.

Lindeman, C. *Birth control and unmarried young women.* New York: Springer, 1974.

MacIntrye, S. *Single and pregnant.* London: Croom Helm, 1977.

Magarick, R. H. Social and emotional aspects of voluntary childlessness in vasectomized childless men. *Dissertation Abstracts,* 1976, 37, 1256A.

Mai, F. M., Munday, R. N., and Rump, E. E. Psychiatric interview comparisons between infertile and fertile couples. *Psychosomatic Medicine,* 1972, 34 (September/October), 431-440.

Marciano, T. D. Male influences on fertility: Needs for research. *The Family Coordinator,* 1979, 28, 561-568.

Marcks, B. R. *Voluntary childless couples: An exploratory study.* M.Sc. dissertation, Syracuse University, 1976.

McCormick, E. P. *Attitudes toward abortion: Experiences of selected black and white women.* Lexington, MA: D. C. Heath, 1975.

Meara, H. Adolescents' use of information about conception and contraception — an exploratory study of cognitive and interactive processes among never married female and male partners who attend birth control clinics for teens. Progress Report (NICHD NOL-HD-82836), September 30, 1980. (Mimeo)

Michel, A. Interaction and family planning in the French urban family. *Demography,* 1967, 4, 615-625.

Miller, W. B. Sexuality, contraception and pregnancy in a high school population. *California Medicine – The Western Journal of Medicine,* August 1973, 14-21.

Miller, W. B. *Some psychological factors predictive of undergraduate sexual and contraceptive behavior.* Paper presented at the Symposium on Teenage Sexuality and Contraceptive Use, American Psychological Association, 84th Annual Convention, Palo Alto, California, September 1976.

Miller, W. B. *The psychology of reproduction.* Final report to the Center for Population Research, NICHD (NOI-HD-82831) by the American Institutes for Research, Palo Alto, California, 1980. (Mimeo)

Misra, B. Correlates of males' attitudes toward family planning. In D. Bogue (Ed.), *Sociological contributions to family planning.* Chicago: Family and Community Study Center, University of Chicago, 1967.

Mitchell, R. E. Husband-wife relations and family planning practices in urban Hong Kong. *Journal of Marriage and the Family,* 1972, 34, 139-146.

Monsour, J. J., and Stewart, B. Abortion and sexual behavior in college women. *American Journal of Orthopsychiatry,* 1973, 43 (October), 804-814.

Morrison, W.A. Attitudes of males toward family planning in a Western Indian village. *Millbank Memorial Fund Quarterly,* 1957, 25, 67-81.

Mukherjee, B. N. The role of husband-wife communication in family planning. *Journal of Marriage and the Family,* 1975, 37, 656-667.

Nair, N. K., and Chow, L. P. Fertility intentions and behavior: Some findings from Taiwan. *Studies in Family Planning,* 1980, 11(7/8), 255-263.

Nason, E. M., and Poloma, M. M. *Voluntarily childless couples: The emergence of a variant lifestyle.* Beverly Hills, CA: Sage Publications, 1976.

Nathanson, C. A. Sex, illness, and medical care. *Social Science and Medicine,* 1977, 11, 13-25.

Ory, M. G. The decision to parent or not: Normative and structural components. *Journal of Marriage and the Family,* 1978, 40 (August), 531-539.

Otero, L. L. The Mexican urbanization process and its implications. *Demography,* 1968, 5, 866-873.

Pannor, R., Massarik, F., and Evans, B. *The unmarried father.* New York: Springer, 1971.

Pearson, J. F. Social and psychological aspects of extramarital first conceptions. *Journal of Biosocial Science,* 1973, 5(4), 453-496.

Peled, T. Psychosocial aspects of abortion in Israel. In H. P. David et al. (Eds.), *Abortion in psychosocial perspective.* New York: Springer, 1978.

Perez-Reyes, M. G. and Falk, R. Follow-up after therapeutic abortion in early adolescence. *Archives of General Psychiatry,* 1973, 28, 120-126.

Phillips, J. F. Continued use of contraception among Philippine family planning acceptors: A multivariate analysis. *Studies in Family Planning,* 1978, 9(7), 182-192.

Platts, H. K. A public adoption agency's approach to natural fathers. *Child Welfare,* 1968, 47, 530-537.

Poffenberger, T., and Poffenberger, S. B. The social psychology of fertility behavior in a village in India. In J. T. Fawcett (Ed.), *Psychological perspectives on population.* New York: Basic Books, 1973.

Polit, D. F. *Contraceptive decision-making in adolescent couples.* Progress Report 3 (NICHD NOI-HD-92835), September 30, 1980. (Mimeo)

Popenoe, P. Motivation of childless marriages. *Journal of Heredity,* 1936, 27 (December), 469-472.

Poti, S.J., Chakraborti, B., and Malaker, C.R. Reliability of data relating to contraceptive practices. In C.V. Kiser (Ed.), *Research in family planning.* Princeton, NJ: Princeton University Press, 1962.

Psychosocial factors in population research. *The male role in contraceptive decision-making and behavior.* Denver: Workshop on Psychosocial Factors, 1980.

Rains, P. *Becoming an unwed mother.* Chicago: Aldine, 1971.

Rainwater, L. *And the poor get children.* Chicago: Quadrangle Books, 1960.

Rainwater, L. *Family design.* Chicago: Aldine, 1965.

Reiss, I.L. *The social context of premarital sexual permissiveness.* New York: Holt, Rinehart, & Winston, 1967.

Renne, K.S. Childlessness, health and marital satisfaction. *Social Biology,* 1976, 23 (Fall), 183-197.

Ritchey, P.N., and Stokes, C.S. Correlates of childlessness and expectations to remain childless. *Social Forces,* 1974, 52 (March), 349-356.

Robbins, J.M. *A forgotten man: The male partner in out-of-wedlock abortion and delivery.* Madison: University of Wisconsin Department of Psychiatry, 1980.

Rosen, R.H. *Decision making on unplanned problem pregnancies.* Unpublished data from NICHD Grant HO-07739. Detroit: Wayne State University, 1976.

Ross, S. *The youth values project.* Washington, D.C.: Population Institute, 1979.

Rothstein, A. Abortion: A dyadic perspective. *American Journal of Orthopsychiatry,* 1977, 47(1), 111-119.

Sabe, M., and Wikler, N. *Up against the clock.* New York: Random House, 1979.

Safilios-Rothschild, C. Family sociology or wives' family sociology? A cross-cultural examination of decision-making. *Journal of Marriage and the Family,* 1969, 31, 290-301.

Scales, P. Males and morals: Teenage contraceptive behavior amid the double standard. *The Family Coordinator,* 1977, 26(3), 211-222.

Scanzoni, J. *Sex roles, life styles and childbearing.* New York: Free Press, 1975.

Schaffer, C., and Pine, F. Pregnancy, abortion and the developmental tasks of adolescence. *American Academy of Child Psychology Journal,* 1972, 11, 511-536.

Schofield, M. *The sexual behavior of young people.* Boston: Little, Brown, 1965.

Shaw, P.C., Funderburk, C., and Franklin, B.J. Investigation of the abortion decision process. *Psychology, a Quarterly Journal of Human Behavior,* 1979, 16(2), 11-19.

Shostak, A.B. Abortion as fatherhood lost: Problems and reforms. *The Family Coordinator,* 1979, 28(4), 569-574.

Silka, L., and Kiesler, S. Couples who choose to be childless. *Family Planning Perspectives,* 1977, 9 (January/February), 16-25.

Sorenson, R.C. *Adolescent sexuality in contemporary america: Personal values and sexual behavior ages 13-19.* New York: World, 1973.

Srinivasan, K., Reddy, P.H., and Raju, K.N.M. From one generation to the next: Changes in fertility, family size preferences, and family planning in an Indian state between 1951 and 1975. *Studies in Family Planning,* 1978, 9(10/11), 258-271.

Stack, C. *All our kin.* New York: Harper & Row, 1974.

Steinhoff, P. G. Premarital pregnancy and the first birth. In W. B. Miller and L. F. Newman (Eds.), *The first child and family formation.* Chapel Hill, NC: Carolina Population Center, 1978.

Sterns, R. S., and Garland, T. N. Factors affecting contraceptive use and nonuse among adolescents. Paper presented at the annual meetings of the National Council on Family Relations. Boston, August 1979.

Stycos, J. M. *Family and fertility in Puerto Rico.* New York: Columbia University Press, 1955.

Stycos J. M. A critique of the traditional planned parenthood approach in under-developed areas. In C. V. Kiser (Ed.), *Research in family planning.* Princeton, NJ: Princeton University Press, 1962.

Stycos, J. M. *Human fertility in Latin America.* Ithaca, NY: Cornell University Press, 1968.

Stycos, J. M. *Ideology, faith and family planning in Latin America.* New York: McGraw-Hill, 1971.

Thompson, L., and Spanier, G. B. Influence of parents, peers, and partners on the contraceptive use of college men and women. *Journal of Marriage and the Family,* 1978, 40, 481-492.

Tobin, P. L., Clifford, W. B., Mustian, R. D., and Davis, A. C. Value of children and fertility behavior in a tri-racial, rural county. *Journal of Comparative Family Studies,* 1975, 6, 46-55.

Townes, B. D., Beach, L. R., Campbell, F. L., and Martin, D. C. Birth planning values and decisions: The prediction of fertility. *Organizational Behavior and Human Performance,* 1976, 15, 99-116.

Trussell, T. J. Economic consequences of teenage childbearing. *Family Planning Perspectives,* 1976, 8, 184-190.

Veenhoven, R. Is there an innate need for children? *European Journal of Social Psychology,* 1974, 4(4), 495-501.

Veevers, J. E. Voluntarily childless wives: An exploratory study. *Sociology and Social Research,* 1973, 57 (April), 356-366.

Veevers, J. E. The life style of voluntarily childless couples. In L. Larson (Ed.), *The Canadian family in comparative perspectives.* Englewood Cliffs, NJ: Prentice-Hall, 1975.

Vincent, C. E. *Unmarried mothers.* New York: Free Press, 1961.

Weinstein, S. A., and Goebel, G. The relationship between contraceptive sex role stereotyping and attitudes toward male contraception among males. *Journal of Sex Research,* 1979, 15(3), 235-242.

Welds, K. *Voluntary childlessness in professional women.* Doctoral dissertation, Harvard University, 1976.

Westoff, C. F., Potter, R. G., Jr., Sagi, P. C., and Mishler, E. G. *Family growth in metropolitan America.* Princeton, NJ: Princeton University Press, 1961.

Whelpton, P. K., Campbell, A. A., and Patterson, J. *Fertility and family planning in the United States.* Princeton, NJ: Princeton University Press, 1966.

Whelpton, P. K., and Kiser, C. V. The comparative influence on fertility of con-traception and impairments of fecundity. *Millbank Memorial Fund Quarterly,* 1948, 26 (April), 182-220.

World Health Organization Task Force on Psychosocial Research in Family Planning and Task Force on Service Research in Family Planning. User preferences for contraceptive methods in India, Korea, the Philippines, and Turkey. *Studies in Family Planning,* 1980, 11(9/10), 267-273.

Zelnik, M., and Kantner, J. F. Sexual and contraceptive experience of young unmarried women in the United States 1976 and 1971. *Family Planning Perspectives,* 1977, 9, 55-71.

Zimmerman, M. K. *Passage through abortion.* New York: Praeger, 1977.

5

Adolescent Contraceptive Use

THE IMPACT OF FAMILY SUPPORT SYSTEMS

Roberta Herceg-Baron and
Frank F. Furstenberg, Jr.

Very little specific information has been generated on the influence that family members exert on adolescent contraceptive behavior. This chapter focuses on the family as a potential source of support for teenage contraceptive use. After first presenting the rationale for studying family influences on adolescent premarital sexual and contraceptive behavior, and a brief review of the research literature, we shall present preliminary findings from an ongoing study of family involvement and support for adolescents seeking birth control from family-planning clinics. The analysis centers on the relationship between the extent of family involvement and the adolescent's subsequent use of contraception.

SPECIAL APPRECIATION is due Al Crawford, Richard Lincoln, Hannah Meara, Barbara Plager, Judy Shea, and Graham Spanier, who have reviewed and commented on drafts of this chapter.

RATIONALE FOR STUDYING
FAMILY INFLUENCES

The essential role that social support systems play in influencing adolescent behavior has long been recognized in the literature on developmental psychology (Elkind, 1967). During this period in their lives, adolescents generally experiment with changing self-concepts and are influenced by family members, other adults, peers, and the media for standards of behavior. Although family members, particularly parents, are frequently assumed to have primary influence over many aspects of their children's socialization, their influence diminishes throughout the teen years and is replaced by the growing influence of peers (Reiss, 1967). In matters of socialization directly related to premarital sexual behavior and contraceptive use, it has been suggested that the family may have relatively little influence on their offspring's behavior when compared to peers. (Thompson and Spanier, 1978; Jorgensen et al., 1980).

Despite these findings, the currently popular wisdom that family involvement is essential for responsible adolescent contraceptive use has not received much empirical scrutiny, particularly among young adolescent populations aged 13-17 years. More research effort needs to be focused specifically on the family's influence on premarital sexual and contraceptive behavior among this group.

A documented decline in the age at first intercourse over the first half of the 1970s (Zelnik and Kantner, 1977) indicated that adolescents were gaining sexual and reproductive experience at earlier ages. At those earlier stages of adolescent development, parental influence may be more evident, since, theoretically, the younger adolescent may still be relatively more receptive to her family as her primary reference group. Under such circumstances, the sexual guidance offered or not offered by an adolescent's parents may become critical to the development of adolescent sexual norms.

Contrary to what might be popularly assumed, the family is not always or necessarily in conflict or competition with the peer group for influence over the adolescent, especially when values are held in common by the two groups. Although peers may influence sexual behavior, as reported in the research literature, the influence is measured in relative terms. The inattentive reader may wrongly infer that because peer or partner influence is stronger, the family's influence is negligible. This inference has not been substantiated by research. Subsequently, the researcher's assumption that the family has a limited role in regulating sexual behavior and contraceptive use has generally diverted research attention away from an examination of the process by which the family learns about the adolescent's sexual and contraceptive behavior and subsequently influences that behavior.

In sum, there has been a tendency to relegate family influence over adolescent sexual and contraceptive behavior to a subordinate role in both research and service efforts, contrary to the popularly held ideal that the family's involvement should be paramount. A fuller understanding of the potential for supportive influences that family members, particularly mothers and sisters, bring to bear on how female adolescents use birth control is needed and could have a significant impact on the way the family is viewed by adolescent health care providers.

REVIEW OF LITERATURE

The Extent of Sexual and Contraceptive Communications within the Family

Parents are not usually a major source of direct sex-related information for adolescents (Thornburg, 1972; Spanier, 1977), although the stated preference in many surveys of both adults and adolescents has been for parental responsibility in sex education (Bennett and Dickinson, 1980; Coughlin and Perales, 1978; General Mills, Inc., 1979). In a comprehensive review of the literature, Fox (1981) concludes that there is little evidence of direct sex communication among family members. If exchange of sex information does occur, it is the mother-daughter dyad that is most significantly involved.

In an extensive study concerning communication between mothers and adolescent daughters about sex and birth control, Fox and Inazu (1980) found that differences in discussion of sex-related topics were associated with the social and structural characteristics of the families studied. Although there were minimal differences by race, household headship, or the mother's educational background in communications about *more* frequently discussed topics, such as menstruation, dating, and boyfriends, differences emerged on *less* widely discussed but more intimate topics, such as sexual morality, intercourse, conception, and birth control. More black mothers than whites discussed sexual intercourse and birth control with their daughters. On the other hand, more white mothers discussed conception with their daughters. Mothers with a college education were more likely to talk about conception and birth control. The topics of sexual intercourse and birth control were discussed less in households where both of the adolescent's biological parents were present than in single-parent households. Family income had a curvilinear relationship to discussions about sexual morality and conception. The mothers with the lowest and highest incomes were less likely to discuss these topics with their daughters than those with moderate incomes. Finally, an examination of mother-daughter discussions by religious background revealed that Catholic mothers were more likely than others to discuss sexuality, morality, and conception but less likely to talk about birth control and sexual intercourse with their daughters. Fox and Inazu suggest that the data shed light on the difficulties existing between mothers and daughters regarding discussion of controversial sex-related topics. Mothers want their daughters to be well-informed; however, mothers do not want to appear to be "pushing" the topics. Daughters want guidance and information but do not want to risk revealing aspects of their own sexual behavior. The "safe" topics for both mothers and daughters were menstruation, dating, and boyfriends. The researchers indicate that since these topics are of general interest to both parent and adolescent but do not necessarily concern intercourse, they may provide the means for initiating discussions of more sensitive sexual topics.

More specific to the use of birth control, another measure of the extent of communication within the family is whether or not parents know about an adolescent's visit to a family-planning clinic for the purpose of receiving contraceptive care. Recent surveys of clinic populations (Torres, 1978; Torres et al., 1980) reveal that just over half of the female adolescents attending family-planning clinics indicate that their parents are aware of their visit. Unfortunately, these studies reveal little about how the parents came to know or how much they supported the adolescent's decision to visit the clinic. Despite the findings that the majority of adolescent family-planning clients report that their parents know about their use of services, these studies also point out that a substantial proportion of the adolescents are receiving care without their parents' knowledge and that some would choose to forego that care, risking unintended pregnancies, rather than reveal to their parents their intentions to visit the clinic.

Both the study of mother-daughter communications and the surveys of parental knowledge about family-planning clinic visits point to the varying extent of communication and knowledge about sex and birth control within the adolescent's family.

Premarital Sexual Behavior and Family Influence

Several studies have linked family influence on the premarital sexual behavior of adolescents with direct family communication about sex. Primarily, the effect of communication with parents about sexual matters seems to have the consequences of delaying the onset of premarital intercourse. A nonrandom survey of male and female college students by Lewis (1973) found that students who received their sex information from sources other than their parents were more likely to have engaged in premarital intercourse than students whose main source of sex education was the parents. Lewis concluded that sex information given primarily by parents would appear to contribute to postponed premarital sexual behavior rather than encourage it.

An analysis of cross-sectional data from a national probability sample of male and female college students by Spanier (1977) revealed that college-aged females whose mothers provided the primary source of sexual information were less likely to have engaged in sexual behavior, whereas gaining information from male friends or independent reading was related to more frequent sexual behavior. This led Spanier to conclude that the sources and content of sex information appear to be important to subsequent sexual behavior, probably due to the attitudes imparted along with the content.

Jessor and Jessor (1975), analyzing longitudinal data, also report on the influence that parents have on the transition of male and female high school and college students from virgin to nonvirgin status, revealing that parental values and support (along with other social and psychological variables) distinguish adolescents who remain virgins from those who initiate sexual activity within a year after being surveyed.

An analysis by Fox and Inazu (1979) showed that mother-daughter discussions about sex encourage responsible sexual behavior among adolescents. They elaborated on their findings by defining the two roles that mothers can and do play when talking to their daughters about sex:

> The first is the role of *protector,* which mothers can assume during the first phase of the sex communication process. . . . The second

role is that of *guide*, in which the mother responds to the daughter's changed sexual status (i.e., non-virgin) by providing more discussion of sex and birth control. The roles are similar in that they both indicate more rather than less communication about sensitive sex-related topics. . . . The *protector* role of the mother seems associated with the postponement of sexual debut by the daughter (at least until 14 or 15 when the daughter was interviewed). Mothers who take on the role of *guide* have the potential for fostering contraceptively responsible behavior on the part of sexually active daughters, either by providing the daughters with necessary information directly or by facilitating the daughters' search for information on their own.

Contraception and Family Influence

The Fox and Inazu (1979) analysis of mother-daughter communications confirms earlier findings by Furstenberg (Furstenberg et al., 1969; Furstenberg, 1971) that parental (particularly maternal) awareness of the adolescent daughter's sexual activity often promotes the latter's use of birth control. In a longitudinal study of adolescent childbearers, Furstenberg noted that most adolescents took great care to conceal their sexual activity from their mothers. The mothers, in turn, feigned ignorance of their daughters' sexual activity, though they openly acknowledged that most of their daughters' peers within the community were involved in sexual relationships. This "mutual agreement of concealment" between mother and daughter typically remained in force until the adolescent became pregnant. However, when this strategy of denial was abandoned as either the daughter or the mother openly acknowledged that sexual relations were occurring, and when some effort to share information about contraception was made, there was a noticeable improvement in the adolescent's use of contraception. Adolescents were more likely to use contraception and more successful in delaying subsequent pregnancies when the mothers knew that they were sexually active and when they talked about using contraception (Furstenberg, 1971).

Support for this finding has appeared in a few other studies as well. Ager et al. (1976), in a study of teenage contraceptors, found that mothers exhibit a strong influence on their adolescent daughters to enroll and continue in a family-planning program. Another study by Ktsanes (1977) found that daughters' perceptions of parental supportiveness contributed to their effective contraceptive practice.

In summary, the literature suggests that direct and well-timed communication by parents about birth-control use may have a beneficial impact on the female adolescent's contraceptive behavior. Since this communication rarely occurs between parents and daughters, but more frequently occurs with partners and peers, it is not surprising that peers and partners appear to be more influential in promoting contraceptive use. The obvious and interesting question arises: What is the impact on adolescent contraceptive behavior when family communication is enhanced? Additional studies of the influence of family support on both male and female adolescent contraceptive practice need to be undertaken. The study described in this chapter is designed to help meet this need by studying a group of young female family-planning clinic attenders who initiate clinic use as adolescents.

METHOD OF STUDY

The Kinship Support Project

An opportunity to study the consequences of enhanced family involvement on female adolescent contraceptive use was provided by the Office of Family Planning in the Bureau of Community Health Services, which late in 1979 funded a service demonstration project to examine and encourage more direct family participation in contraceptive programs for adolescents. The Kinship Project, as it has come to be called, is a service delivery research project conducted in six family-planning agencies affiliated with the Family Planning Council of Southeastern Pennsylvania.

The adolescents in this study were recruited from a variety of family-planning clinic sites, including hospitals, Planned Parenthood affiliates, and community-based programs. All clinics were located in the metropolitan Philadelphia area. The adolescents were randomly assigned to one of three service groups: family support, periodic support, or a control group. Adolescents assigned to the family support group were offered a series of counseling sessions with trained counselors. These adolescents were encouraged to bring at least one family member with them, to share problems relating to sex and contraception. The aims of these sessions were to deal with potential conflicts, to reduce the atmosphere of secrecy, and to devise strategies for rendering assistance to the adolescents in the event such aid was required. Adolescents in the periodic support group received frequent telephone contacts by trained research assistants, who talked with the adolescents about their use of birth control but did not provide any specific encouragement to communicate with their families. Adolescents in the control group received no additional support services aside from those provided through the conventional services offered in family-planning programs for teenagers.

The effects of receiving these services on the adolescent's use of birth control will be considered in subsequent studies, since our sample here is too small for service group comparisons. In this chapter we shall draw on information collected in the evaluation of the Kinship Project to examine the relationship between extent of family knowledge and communication about the adolescent's use of birth control and her subsequent use of contraception.

Data Collection Procedures

During the period from January 1980 through July 1981, data on close to 500 nonpregnant female adolescent clients (under 18 years of age) were collected through structured, face-to-face interviews conducted by trained research assistants during the adolescent's first birth-control visit to the participating agency.

Adolescents participating in the study were interviewed by telephone two additional times to assess the impact of changing family communication patterns on contraceptive use. The first of these follow-up interviews was scheduled at six months after the initial visit but actually occurred any time between the fifth and ninth months. Currently we are midway through the second round of data collection. Therefore, the results reported here, which use data from both the initial interview and the six-month follow-up, represent preliminary findings on a partial sample of adolescents for whom we have completed two interviews. The final follow-up interviews, scheduled to occur eighteen months after the initial visit, commenced in July 1981. Cooperation on this study has been excellent, and follow-up interview rates range from 85 to 95 percent, depending on the clinic in which the initial interviews took place.

The two interviews on which this study is based contain questions about family members' knowledge of the clinic visit, family communication about sex and birth control, contraceptive use during the interval preceding the first follow-up, and demographic characteristics.

SAMPLE CHARACTERISTICS

Demographic Information

Of the 208 respondents whose initial and six-month interviews were available for data analysis, 51 percent were white, 49 percent were black, and one respondent was of Hispanic origin. All were under 18 years of age at the time of the initial interview. Approximately one-third were 17 years old, one-third were 16, and the remaining one-third were between 13 and 15 years old inclusive. Almost all of these adolescents (90 percent) indicated that they were full-time students.

Just over half of the respondents (52 percent) lived in households where both a biological or stepparent mother and father were present. Of these, 85 percent said they lived with their biological mothers and 52 percent said they lived with the biological fathers. The educational level of the adolescents' guardians varied considerably. Nearly one-third (31 percent) of the mothers had not completed high school; just under half (49 percent) had gone as far as completing high school; one-fifth (20 percent) had some advanced college or technical training. The fathers were more highly educated. One-quarter (26 percent) had not completed high school; 44 percent were high school graduates, and nearly one-third (30 percent) had had some advanced technical or college-level training.

The six agencies participating in this study were selected in an effort to recruit adolescents from a cross-section of families who utilize federally funded family-planning programs. The partial sample surveyed for this chapter provides such a cross-section but is too small to analyze further by age, race, and family socioeconomic status.

Sexual and Contraceptive Background

Despite the fact that 86 percent of these girls were nonvirgins, very few of the respondents had had previous contact with either a family-planning or a private physician in order to get birth control. Of the adolescents who were sexually active, 75 percent had had intercourse by the time they were 15 years old. Sexual activity among these teens was infrequent and use of effective methods of birth control sporadic. In the four weeks prior to their initial clinic visit, 31 percent had not had intercourse at all, and 43 percent had had intercourse once a week or less frequently. Many of the adolescents (or their partners) were predisposed toward preventing a pregnancy and had made some effort to use a method of birth control; however, few of the teens had ever used medically prescribed methods of contraception prior to their first clinic visit. They most likely mentioned withdrawal (46 percent) or rhythm (24 percent) as the method of birth control they had previously practiced. Moreover, 46 percent of the adolescents reported that they did not use any method of contraception the last time they had had intercourse. The adolescents' episodic sexual encounters, coupled with their sporadic use of birth control, may account for the fact that 27 percent of them had experienced a previous pregnancy and 64 percent reported having had a "pregnancy scare."

Nearly three-quarters of the adolescents (74 percent) had come to the clinic for their initial visit accompanied by someone. The majority of the accompanied adolescents (58 percent) had come with one or more girlfriends and another 12 percent with boyfriends. There were 15 percent who came with their mothers, and the remaining 15 percent came in the company of sisters or other relatives.

RESULTS OF THE STUDY

Changing Patterns of Family Communication about Sex and Birth Control

A logical place to begin an investigation of the level of family support for contraceptive use is to examine the extent of communications adolescents have with other family members about sex and birth control. Table 5.1 shows that 74 percent of the adolescents were able to identify at least one family member with whom they had discussed sex and birth control at the time of the initial interview. At the six-month follow-up, communication increased slightly, to 83 percent. Clearly, the majority of these adolescents can identify some family member(s) with whom they talk about sexual matters, although our data do not reveal the extent or content of the discussions. Not surprisingly, sisters and mothers are the most frequently mentioned family members at the initial interview, with sisters being mentioned somewhat more often than mothers; they are named by 49 percent and 40 percent of the respondents, respectively. At the time of the six-month follow-up, the tendency to share confidences with

TABLE 5.1   Family Communication about Sex and Birth Control

| Family Member | *Percentage Involved in Talking with Family Member* | | |
	Initial Interview	*6-Month Follow-Up*	*Number*
Anyone	74	83	208
Mother	40	36	200
Father	4	2	157
Sister(s)	49	64	110
Brother(s)	4	3	122

sisters is even more noticeable. While mothers are mentioned by only 36 percent of the adolescents, sisters at this point are considered as confidantes by nearly two-thirds of the teens (64 percent). We find that fathers and brothers are least likely to be identified as nuclear family members with whom the adolescents talk.

In an effort to understand the shifting patterns of communication suggested here, we selected for further examination the 108 respondents in our sample who indicated that their mothers and at least one adolescent sister were present in the household. As shown in Table 5.2, at the time of the initial interview just under one-third of the respondents (29 percent) admitted to not being able to talk to either their mothers or their sisters about birth control. Few adolescents (14 percent) could talk to both mothers and sisters. Over one-third of the adolescents (35 percent) identified only sisters as confidantes, while just over one-fifth of the teens (22 percent) could talk only with their mothers. By comparison, when the same question was asked six months later, the respondents were more likely to mention sisters only (54 percent), and the number of adolescents singling out their mothers as their only confidantes dropped by half. Approximately one respondent in four was unable to talk to either her mother or her sister(s).

Apparently, then, confidences within the family network change over time and, in our study, this change primarily involves the sisters engaging in closer confidences with the respondents rather than the respondents expanding their involvement with their mothers. It is also evident that a substantial minority of respondents have better communication with their mothers than with sisters. Yet, a significant proportion of adolescents do not perceive either their mothers or their sisters as family members with whom they can discuss sex-related topics. The diversity of support patterns revealed by our data

TABLE 5.2   Mother and Sister Communication about Sex and Birth
Control (N = 108)

Family Member	Percentage Involved in Talking with Mothers and Sisters	
	Initial Interview	*6-Month Follow-Up*
Neither mother nor sister talk	29	24
Mother only talks	22	11
Sister only talks	35	54
Both mother and sister talk	14	11

TABLE 5.3   Family Member Knowledge of Clinic Visit

Family Member	Percentage Knowing about Clinic Visit		
	Initial Interview	*6-Month Follow-Up*	*Number*
Anyone	61	82	208
Mother	42	62	200
Father	12	25	157
Sister(s)	46	57	110
Brother(s)	8	16	122

suggests that no single model can be designed sufficiently to facilitate communication within the family.

Changing Patterns of Family Communication about the Clinic Visit

One would surmise that the adolescents who talk with a family member would also be more likely to share information about their intentions to use the clinic. When we examine the data from the initial interview to determine who in the family knows of the visit to the clinic (Table 5.3), the proportions for individual family members are similar to the data on family communication from the initial interview (as presented in Table 5.1), although slightly more fathers and brothers know about the visit than the respondents indicate as persons with whom they can usually talk. However, by the six-month follow-up some interesting differences emerge. Not surprisingly, more family members know about the clinic visit by the six-month follow-up than knew originally, regardless of their familial relation-

TABLE 5.4   Mother and Sister Knowledge about Clinic Visit (N = 108)

Family Member	Percentage Knowing about Clinic Visit	
	Initial Interview	*6-Month Follow-Up*
Neither mother nor sister knows	37	18
Mother only knows	17	25
Sister only knows	21	24
Both mother and sister know	25	33

ship with the adolescent. The proportions of fathers and brothers knowing double (from 12 to 25 percent and from 8 to 16 percent, respectively), while the proportion of mothers knowing increases by half (from 42 to 62 percent). The chances of one or more sisters knowing of the clinic visit increase slightly, from 46 to 57 percent.

Interestingly, except for sisters, the increase in knowledge about the clinic visit is not reflected in a similar increase in the adolescents' ability to talk with those individual family members about sex and birth control, as described in the previous section.

Since these two interviews unfortunately do not contain information about how the family members learn of the clinic visit, we are limited in the conclusions we can draw from this disparity, except to say that the adolescents in our study do not equate a family member's *knowledge* about the clinic visit with increased and comfortable *communication* about sex and birth control. This topic will be explored in greater detail in our eighteen-month follow-up, which provides more specific data on how family members learn about the clinic visit.

Again, looking at the data available on adolescents living in households with both mothers and sister(s) present (Table 5.4), we find that half of the respondents who had told neither family member at the time of the initial visit had shared this information with the mother, the sister(s), or both by the six-month follow-up. The data indicate that by the second interview 58 percent of the mothers know about the visit, compared with 42 percent at the initial interview, representing a 38 percent increase. The proportion of sisters knowing increased 24 percent, from 46 percent to 57 percent respectively.

Therefore, from our findings it appears that in the six months following their clinic visit, adolescents tend to open up communication with their sisters about the general topics of sex and birth control, but the mothers are more frequently the ones who learn about the visit to the clinic.

Before we examine the effects that communication and knowledge about the clinic visit have on the respondents' use of contraception, it is important to pause and consider the implications that changes in family communications and knowledge about the clinic visit have for the design of family-planning services. Since communication patterns within the family are likely to change over the time interval of six months from the first clinic visit, the family-planning counselor could be instrumental in working with the adolescent, not only to identify family members who presently support her, but also to help the adolescent to expand her vision of support by considering potential allies that may in the near future emerge among other family members. According to our data, these family members are most likely to be sisters; however, there is some value in encouraging the adolescent to examine her relationship with her mother more closely, since this is the one family member more than others who is likely to learn about the clinic visit later. In working with the adolescent in this fashion, the counselor can help her to deal constructively with a mother who "finds out" or can facilitate the daughter's efforts to broach the topic with her mother prior to her "finding out." In some cases, these efforts on the part of the counselor might eventually evolve into counseling sessions with the mother-daughter pair. Discussions about the clinic visit could be used as the point of departure in efforts to build support for and increase effective communication about sex and birth control between mother and daughter. It is likely, although we will not have data to examine our suspicions until we complete the eighteen-month follow-up, that adolescents who "volunteer" the information or have been "transparent" about their clinic visits in the hopes of initiating communication with their mothers will gain more support for contraceptive use from having communicated this than will adolescents whose mothers have "found them out" only after protracted periods of careful and conscious concealment of the information on the part of the daughter.

BIRTH-CONTROL USE AS IT RELATES TO FAMILY COMMUNICATION

By the time of the six-month follow-up, most of the respondents in our study (66 percent) could be classified as effective contraceptors.[1]

TABLE 5.5   Effect of Family Communication on Birth Control Use at 6-Month Follow-Up

	Percentage Who Are Effective Users at 6-Month Follow-Up							
	Initial Interview				*6-Month Follow-Up*			
Family Member	*Talks*	*(N)*	*Doesn't Talk*	*(N)*	*Talks*	*(N)*	*Doesn't Talk*	*(N)*
Anyone	69	(147)	59	(51)	68	(165)	58	(33)
Mother	66	(77)	65	(114)	75	(67)	60	(124)
Sister(s)	65	(52)	60	(53)	61	(67)	66	(38)

Comparing contraceptive behavior in the time previous to the clinic visit with the one month previous to the six-month interview, we note a significant increase in effective use (23 percent compared to 72 percent). A central question in this chapter concerns the association between the adolescents' ability to contracept effectively at the time of their follow-up interviews and the communication pattern they had established with family members both at the time they first came to the clinic and six months later. Table 5.5 reveals that although there is a slight tendency for the more effective users to be adolescents who can talk with a family member and with a mother specifically, the differences are not great and certainly not statistically significant.

Similarly, we did not observe much discrimination among effective users when we tested for associations between use of and family knowledge about the clinic visit (Table 5.6). Adolescents who had told no one in their families about the clinic visit were as likely to be using birth control effectively as those who had told someone.

Subsequent analyses that examine combinations of family-member communication about sex and birth control and/or family-member knowledge of the clinic visit also yield no significant support for our hypothesis that enhanced family communication is associated with the adolescent's ability to use contraception effectively.

In any event, what remains striking about our analyses at six months is that, regardless of family involvement behaviors, there is a significant proportion of adolescents (approximately one-third) who are having difficulty practicing effective contraception, despite the fact that they have recently enrolled in a contraceptive program.

DISCUSSION AND CONCLUSIONS

The data suggest that, contrary to our expectation, family communication about sex and birth control is not associated with effective

TABLE 5.6   Effect of Family Knowledge about Clinic Visit on
Birth-Control Use

	Percentage Who Are Effective Users at 6-Month Follow-Up							
	Initial Interview				*6-Month Follow-Up*			
Family Member	*Knows*	*(N)*	*Doesn't Know*	*(N)*	*Knows*	*(N)*	*Doesn't Know*	*(N)*
Anyone	69	(118)	62	(80)	67	(162)	61	(36)
Mother	65	(77)	66	(114)	67	(117)	64	(74)
Sister(s)	65	(46)	61	(59)	62	(60)	64	(45)

contraceptive use, nor is there a relationship between family knowledge about the teen's visit to the clinic and effective contraceptive use. Although we note changes in family communication patterns and knowledge about the clinic visit over a six-month period, the proportion of effective users remains about the same, whether or not the family members know about the visit or can talk with the girls about sex and birth control (approximately 60 to 70 percent of the girls in each group are effective users). It is possible that our measures of family factors are too crude and that the strength of family relationships (or closeness) is an intervening factor that may qualify the content and tone of the discussions about sex and birth control. In a similar fashion, how the family members came to learn about the clinic visit may qualify our measure of family knowledge about the visit. A third possible explanation for the absence of any strong association between family involvement and birth-control use is that six months is too short a time in which to gain a reliable measure of contraceptive behavior for these adolescents, since this "novice" period may not be typical of long-term contraceptive behavior patterns.

Based on data presented here, we must conclude that the family's involvement in adolescent contraceptive use is a complex phenomenon that must be viewed as having the potential to change over time and among family members. We discovered strong evidence that changes take place in family communication during the interval between the clinic visit and six-month follow-up. Overall, there is an increase in the amount of communication as teenagers become more sexually experienced. However, our data suggest that the increase in communication does not inevitably lead to greater family support (in particular, support from the adolescent's mother). Indeed, there is some indication that communication with the mother may drop off or become more oblique in some cases, as teenagers become more involved in their sexual relationships. This may result not because the mother is disapproving, but because over time adolescents gradually become more involved with their peers than with their parents.

The philosophy behind the Kinship Project was to test one family-oriented model for modifying design and delivery of family-planning services to adolescents, which have traditionally been pervaded by an ethos of individualism wherein services are directed to individuals with little regard for the social context in which those individuals exist. While we were unable to test for treatment effects in this study, at the same time, our analyses shed some doubt upon the unqualified assertion that family involvement will be the elixir for promoting responsible and effective contraceptive use among adolescents. Certainly, communication per se is not associated with effective contraceptive use. Furthermore, interventions on behalf of the adolescent by her family will have to account for the great diversity of family constellations within which communication about sex and birth control occur.

Given the exploratory nature of efforts that are currently under way to involve the family voluntarily and to assess the family's impact, it is more sensible for policymakers and family-planning program administrators to promote the flexibility necessary for further experimentation and evaluation of family-oriented programs, rather than succumb to current political pressures to mandate rigid solutions, such as parental consent or notification, that have not yet been developed or tested.

It is also important and practical to note that in a climate of decreased funding for federally supported health programs such as family-planning services, there will be fewer opportunities for programs to develop the staff training needed and to expand programs necessary for providing meaningful services to both adolescents and their families.

NOTE

1. Those sample members whom we designated as "effective contraceptors" are (1) those who used a reliable method of birth control (such as the Pill, IUD, diaphragm, foam and/or condoms) "all of the time" during periods of sexual activity between the initial and follow-up interval, and (2) those respondents who met the above-mentioned criteria with the exception that they used these methods less than all of the time during one month. In most of the later instances ($N = 19$), the month

missed was the first month, during which there was often a lag or complication in the provision of a method of contraception.

REFERENCES

Ager, J., Shea, F., and Agronow, S. *Comparisons of participants and dropout from a teen contraceptive program.* Paper presented at the Eighty-Fourth Annual Convention of the American Psychological Association, Washington, D.C., 1976.

Bennett, S. M., and Dickinson, W. B. Student-parent rapport and parent involvement in sex, birth control, and venereal disease education. *Journal of Sex Research*, 1980, 16, 114-130.

Coughlin, D. J., and Perales, C. A. Family planning and the teenager; A service delivery assessment. Report to the Secretary of Health, Education, and Welfare, New York, November, 1978.

Elkind, D. Egocentrism in adolescence. *Child Development*, 1967, 38, 1025-1034.

Fox, G. L. The mother-daughter relationship and sexual socialization structure: A research review. *Family Relations*, 1980, 29, 21-28.

Fox, G. L. The family's role in adolescent sexual behavior. In T. Ooms (Ed.), *Teenage pregnancy in a family context: Implications in policy.* Philadelphia: Temple University Press, 1981.

Fox, G. L. and Inazu, J. K. *The effect of mother-daughter communication on daughter's sexual and contraceptive knowledge and behavior.* Paper presented at the annual meeting of the Population Association of America, Philadelphia, 1979.

Fox, G. L., and Inazu, J. K. Mother-daughter communication about sex. *Family Relations*, 1980, 29, 347-352.

Furstenberg, F. F. Birth control experience among pregnant adolescents: The process of unplanned parenthood. *Social Problems*, 1971, 19, 192-203.

Furstenberg, F. F., Markowitz, M., and Gordis, L. Birth control knowledge and attitudes among unmarried pregnant adolescents. *Journal of Marriage and the Family*, 1969, 30, 34-42.

General Mills, Inc. *General Mills American family report, 1978-79.* Minneapolis, MN: General Mills, Inc., 1979.

Jessor, S. L., and Jessor, R. Transition from virginity to nonvirginity among youth: A social psychological study over time. *Developmental Psychology*, 1975, 11, 473-484.

Jorgensen, S. R., King, S. L., Torrey, B. A. Dyadic and social network influences on adolescent exposure to pregnancy risk. *Journal of Marriage and the Family*, 1980, 42, 141-155.

Ktsanes, V. Assessment of contraception by teenagers. Final report to NICHD (1HD-52833), 1977.

Lewis, R. A. Parents and peers: Socialization agents in the coital behavior of young adults. *Journal of Sex Research*, 1973, 9, 156-170.

Reiss, I. L. *The social context of premarital sexual permissiveness.* New York: Holt, Rinehart, and Winston, 1967.

Spanier, G. B. Sources of sex information and premarital sexual behavior. *Journal of Sex Research*, 1977, 13, 2, 73-88.

Thompson, L., and Spanier, G. B. Influence of parents, peers and partners on the contraceptive use of college men and women. *Journal of Marriage and the Family,* 1978, 40, 481-492.

Thornburg, H. D. A comparative study of sex information sources. *Journal of School Health,* 1972, 42, 88-91.

Torres, A. Does your mother know . . .? *Family Planning Perspectives,* 1978, 10, 280-282.

Torres, A., Forrest, J. D., and Eisman, S. Telling parents: Clinic policies and adolescents' use of family planning and abortion services. *Family Planning Perspectives,* 1980, 12, 284-292.

Zelnik, M., and Kantner, J. Sexual and contraceptive experience of young unmarried women in the U.S., 1976 and 1971. *Family Planning Perspectives,* 1977, 9, 55-71.

6

Motivational Bases of Childbearing Decisions

Frederick L. Campbell,
Brenda D. Townes,
and Lee Roy Beach

For more than three decades, population scientists have pursued, without much success, that Questing Beast, the psychological determinants of fertility. But like the mythical King Pellinore, we seem to find only the beasts' fewmets (White, 1939). In recent years, there have been new calls to the chase (Fawcett, 1973; Pohlman, 1969; Newman and Thompson, 1976), and the pursuit has required new strategies. One such strategy is the application of decision-theoretic models to the study of childbearing. In this chapter we discuss the use of selected sociological and psychological approaches to the study of fertility and then describe an application of a decision-theoretic

THIS PROJECT was supported by Research Grant HD-07225-01 A from the National Institute of Child Health and Human Development, Center for Population Research, and by NICHD Center Grant HD-09397-01 to the Center for Studies in Demography and Ecology, University of Washington.

model, subjective expected utility, to the study of the motivational bases of birth-planning decisions.

SOCIOLOGICAL AND PSYCHOLOGICAL APPROACHES

Failure to isolate the psychological determinants of fertility has been well documented. More than 35 years ago, the pioneering Indianapolis Study undertook to discover the social and psychological factors associated with fertility (Whelpton and Kiser, 1946-1958). This was the largest survey of fertility behavior undertaken up to that time; it involved interviews with 1,444 white Protestant couples in which both husband and wife had at least an eighth-grade education. There were five major categories in relation to which hypotheses were developed. One of them concerned the personal characteristics of the respondents: feeling of personal inadequacy, feelings that children interfered with personal freedom, ego-centered interest in children, fear of pregnancy, tendency to plan, interest in religion, adherence to traditions, and conformity to group patterns (Kiser and Whelpton, 1953). The yield from these psychological variables was small, indeed so small that in looking back on the effort, Kiser and Whelpton (1958: 318) concluded that "for the present, the chief lesson to be emphasized concerns the generally closer relationship of fertility to broad social factors (including the economic) than to psychological factors."

This lesson did not take well, however, for it was easy to see where things might have gone wrong. The adequacy of the concepts, problems of measurement, and the absence of a clearly defined behavioral target were all discussed. In 1954, a study of family growth in metropolitan America (the Princeton Study) was undertaken, in part, to reappraise the importance of psychological factors (Westoff et al., 1961). This study was based on interview data obtained from an initial panel of 1,165 white women who lived in one of the largest metropolitan areas in the United States and who had recently given birth to a second child. Considerable attention was given to the conceptualization of the psychological variables, and the main battery consisted of generalized manifest anxiety, need for nurturance, compulsiveness, tolerance of ambiguity, cooperativeness, and need for achievement. The measurement of these concepts was as good as the state of the art allowed and probably could not be much improved upon today, given the constraints of survey research. Finally, the question under study was restricted to the relatively straightforward decision about whether to have a third child. At the conclusion of the first phase of this longitudinal study, only very low correlations were found between the psychological variables and the two fertility measures under analysis, number of children desired and family-planning success. In the second phase of the study no significant associations were found between the psychological variables and the subsequent bearing of a third child (Westoff et al., 1963). Once again, social and economic factors dominated psychological factors affecting fertility.

Three other major surveys of nationally representative samples were conducted in the following decade. These were the 1955 and 1960 Growth of American Families (GAF) studies (Freedman et al., 1959; Whelpton et al., 1966) and the 1965 National Fertility Study (see Westoff and Ryder, 1969). Results from these studies established even more firmly the influential importance of structural-behavioral factors on contraceptive use, fertility expectations, and childbearing.

THE LINGERING QUESTION

We are left then with the question of what determines fertility at the personal level. What we have learned about fertility at the aggregate level does not seem to help. For example, responses to the question of desired family size, when treated as group averages, are good predictors of aggregate fertility. Yet, the evidence from longitudinal studies indicates that such responses are poor predictors of individuals' subsequent childbearing (Bumpass and Westoff, 1969, 1970; Goldberg et al., 1959; Westoff et al., 1957; Westoff et al., 1963). Similarly, knowledge of the social and economic correlates of fertility does not necessarily explain individual behavior. It has been repeatedly pointed out that to know that religious affiliation or class standing is differentially related to fertility does not answer the question of *why* this should be so (see Fawcett, 1974; Pohlman, 1969; Rainwater, 1965). More recently, Jaccard and Davidson (1976: 330) have said that "if we are to understand fertility-related behavior, it is clear that we must not only describe variation in fertility but also determine the process by which social and economic variables operate through psychological variables to influence desired family size."

DECISION-THEORETIC EXPLANATIONS
OF FERTILITY

Recently, attempts have been made to conceptualize fertility as the outgrowth of a rational decision-making process. Assume for the moment that individuals are capable of making rational choices with respect to their own childbearing. Next, accept the observation that there is always a set of rewards and costs associated with the decision to have a, or another, child. Assume further that individuals make choices that tend to maximize their rewards and minimize their costs. It then would follow that if individuals had the means to implement a fertility decision (contraceptive effectiveness), they would, barring unforeseen events (illness, dissolution of the reproductive relationship), follow a course of action that would maximize their expected rewards and minimize their expected costs. This idea, in various forms, has been used to explain fertility at two different levels of analysis. Economists have used decision theory to explain variation in fertility rates at the aggregate level, such as differences in completed family size among social classes (see Easterlin, 1967). Psychologists have used variants of decision theory to explain the way individuals come to make particular fertility decisions (Adler, 1979).

Recently, a number of attempts have been made to apply decision-theoretic models (or related concepts) to fertility-related behavior. These attempts include the prediction of attitudes toward birth control (Crawford, 1973; Insko et al., 1970; Kothandapani, 1971), contraceptive use (Davidson and Jaccard, 1976), abortion (Smetana and Adler, 1979), maternal employment (Beckman, 1978; Beckman and Houser, 1979), desired family size (Kirchner and Seaver, 1977), the intention to have a particular number of children (Inazu et al., 1974; Werner et al., 1975), and the decision to have another child (Townes et al., 1980).

The differences between the models used in these various studies are subtle. For each, however, the basic assumptions concerning rational calculation of utilities and maximization of gain and/or minimization of loss remain roughly the same as those used in economic utility models. A major difference in studying decision-making at the individual level is the need to move from measurement of objective costs and benefits, which are determined by the nature of the social structure and the workings of the economy, to measurement of subjective costs and benefits, which are based on the individual's perception of gains and losses. To accomplish this goal, the present study employed a subjective expected utility model to investigate motivations underlying fertility decisions among couples of varying parity.

METHODS

Subjects

Subjects in the study were 199 married couples, including 51 with no children, 50 with one child, 51 with two children, and 47 with three or four children. Criteria for inclusion in the study were: current use of a contraceptive, no history of infertility or adoption, no previous sterilization, Caucasian, non-Catholic, married, and a reasonable likelihood of continued residence in the Seattle metropolitan area for at least two years. Subjects were recruited from educational and religious organizations. They were primarily highly educated and middle-class (Townes et al., 1980).

Procedures

The Hierarchy of Birth Planning Values (Hierarchy) was administered to husbands and wives in separate rooms.[1] The Hierarchy (see Table 6.1) was constructed to contain a comprehensive list of hierarchically arranged values associated with birth-planning decisions. The development of the instrument and detailed methods of scoring are described in earlier articles (Beach et al., 1979, 1976). To summarize briefly, the subjects first read over the Hierarchy to become familiar with its contents. Then they examined more closely the lower-level categories 1-4. (These categories consisted of the category titles listed in Table 6.1 plus some exemplars that served to define them more specifically.) Next they assigned a+ to the category if its contents argued for having a child and a− if the contents argued against having a child. Then they assigned relative important ratings to the four categories by dividing 100 points among them in proportion to their importance in the subject's deliberations about whether to have a child. Finally, they estimated the probability that the considerations in each category would indeed occur if a child were born.

TABLE 6.1   Hierarchy of Birth-Planning Values

  I. Values Centered on Self and Spouse
     A. Personal identity
        1. Physical aspects of having a baby
        2. Growth and maturity
        3. Self-concept
        4. Educational and vocational values
     B. Parenthood
        5. Caring for the child
        6. Parents' role in education and training a child
        7. Parent-child relationships
     C. Well-being of family
        8. Material well-being of family
        9. Nonmaterial well-being of family
       10. Well-being of self and spouse
       11. Well-being of the marriage
 II. Values Centered on Children
     A. Family Characteristics
       12. Family size and sexes of children
       13. Ages of parents
     B. Health and well-being of children
       14. Sibling relationships
       15. Prospective child
       16. Effects of society on child
III. Values Centered on Significant Others
     A. Family
       17. Relationships with relatives
       18. Family traditions
     B. 19. Friends
     C. 20. Society

This procedure was done for each of the groupings of arabic-numbered lower-level categories in the hierarchy (1-4, 5-7, 8-11, and so on). Then 100 points were divided among the groupings of second-level categories (IA-IC, IIA and IIB, IIIA-IIIC) to indicate their relative importance. Finally, yet another 100 points were divided among the top-level categories (I, II, III).

Multiplying the proportions of importance (utility) points down the hierarchy from the top level (roman numerals) to the lowest level (arabic numerals) gives the relative utility of the twenty lowest-level categories. These are then weighted by their probabilities of occurrence (that is, multiplied by the probability). Then, by appropriately affixing the + and − signs, one arrives at a subjective expected utility (SEU) for each of the twenty categories. The sum of the positive (+)

SEUs for an individual gives the degree of overall positive expectations about the effects of having a (another) child (SEU+ +SEU- =1.00). It is this aggregate that is used to predict the decision: It is called the total SEU+. In what follows we will deal with both the total SEU+ and the twenty level SEU+'s. Group differences are evaluated by univariate and multivariate analyses of variance; two-tailed significance levels were used throughout.[2]

RESULTS

Family Size and Childbearing Values

The first question to be considered is the effect of family size on the perceived costs and benefits husbands and wives associate with having another child. In doing so, there is a separate analysis for husbands and wives. The total SEU+ scores were compared by analysis of variance for the four group comparisons and by the t test for the two group comparisons. SEU+ scores at the twenty-variable level were compared across parities by means of linear discriminant analysis. The results, shown in Table 6.2, reveal that husbands with no children differ in values associated with birth-planning decisions from those with one or more children. Husbands with at least one child, however, do not differ in fertility-relevant values as parity increases. By contrast, among married women there is a more articulated set of values associated with birth planning at each parity up to the second parity. Women with two or more children did not differ from one another. Wives with no children differ from those with one or more children, and married women with one child differ from those with two and three or more children in their subjective expected utilities associated with continued childbearing. The next, and most interesting, question is the nature of these differences.

Motivations For and Against Childbearing

The total SEU+ scores for husbands and wives by parity is plotted in Figure 6.1. A score above 50 implies a positive motivation toward further childbearing, a score below 50 implies a negative motivation toward further childbearing, and a score around 50 implies ambivalence. Note that husbands and wives are quite similar, within parity, in their overall motivation for childbearing. The figure shows

TABLE 6.2 Across Parity Comparisons of Subjective Expected Utility Scores for (a) Males and (b) Females

Sex	Variable	Parity						
		0,1,2,3/4	0,1	1,2	2,3/4	0,2	0,3/4	1,3/4
(a) Males	Total SEU+	$F = 1.60$ df = 3 p = n.s.	$t = -.69$ df = 96.82 p = n.s.	$t = 1.98$ df = 98.39 p < .05	$t = -1.47$ df = 95.99 p = n.s.	$t = 1.45$ df = 95.24 p = n.s.	$t = -.13$ df = 91.68 p = n.s.	$t = .51$ df = 94.56 p = n.s.
	Twenty-level SEU+	$\chi^2 = 91.39$ df = 60 p < .01	$\chi^2 = 44.17$ df = 20 p < .001	$\chi^2 = 20.54$ df = 20 p = n.s.	$\chi^2 = 20.27$ df = 20 p = n.s.	$\chi^2 = 50.58$ df = 20 p < .001	$\chi^2 = 38.83$ df = 20 p < .01	$\chi^2 = 10.77$ df = 20 p = n.s.
(b) Females	Total SEU+	$F = 4.32$ df = 3 p < .01	$t = -2.24$ df = 98.96 p < .05	$t = 3.37$ df = 94.33 p < .001	$t = -.42$ df = 95.37 p = n.s.	$t = 1.35$ df = 96.02 p = n.s.	$t = .87$ df = 88.89 p = n.s.	$t = 2.82$ df = 87.20 p < .02
	Twenty-level SEU+	$\chi^2 = 117.73$ df = 60 p < .001	$\chi^2 = 54.62$ df = 20 p < .001	$\chi^2 = 30.98$ df = 20 p < .001	$\chi^2 = 20.66$ df = 20 p = n.s.	$\chi^2 = 46.82$ df = 20 p < .001	$\chi^2 = 38.96$ df = 20 p < .01	$\chi^2 = 33.84$ df = 20 p < .05

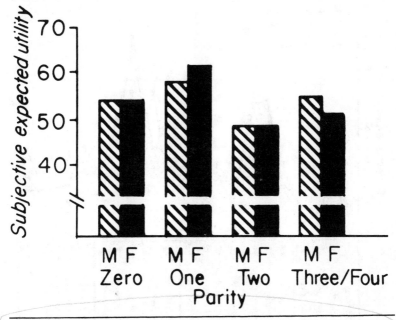

Figure 6.1 Total Subjected and Expected Utility Scores Plotted for Males and Females by Parity

that couples who have no children are ambivalent about having the first child. Couples with one child are quite positive about having a second child, while those with two children are negative about having a third child. Those with three or four children are once again ambivalent about continued childbearing, with the husbands slightly more positive than the wives.

The components of the overall motivation are shown in Figures 6.2, for males, and Figure 6.3, for females. When examining Figures 6.2 and 6.3, remember that high scores indicate maximizing subjective expected utility by having a (another) child; low scores indicate minimizing costs by not having a (another) child.

In Figures 6.2 and 6.3, we see that both costs and rewards of childbearing are recognized. For both men and women across all parity groups, the primary motivations for childbearing are the opportunity to establish a close affiliative relationship with another human being (7: parent/child relationships) and the opportunity to participate in the education and training of the child (6: child's education). The major deterrents (costs) to childbearing are the negative impact of a

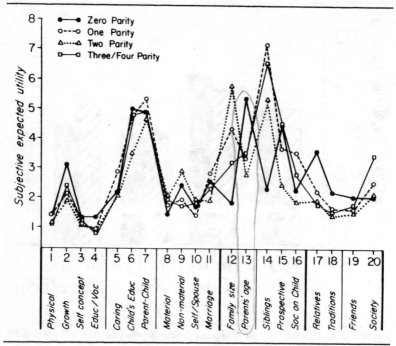

Figure 6.2 Mean Scores by Parity of Male Subjects on the 20-Level Subjective Expected Utility Scores

child upon attainment of parents' educational and vocational goals (4: education/vocation) and the material well-being of the family (8: material). There are, however, some specific rewards and costs associated with each parity level as well as these communalities.

As couples ponder the decision to have a first child, their age at the time of childbearing (13: parents' age) is a major motivation for having a child. It is important to have the first child while they are young. In this they differ significantly from men (F = 3.41; d.f. = 3,195; p <.05) and women (F = 4.63; d.f. = 3,195; ; p <.01) who already have one or more children. A second motivation for having the first child is the expectation of both husbands (F = 4.46; d.f. = 3,195; p <.01) and wives (F = 5.71; d.f. = 3,195; p <.01) that producing a grandchild for their parents and a niece or nephew for their brothers or sisters will establish, maintain, and enhance affiliation with their parents and other family members (17: relatives). Here, then, we see the effects of socialization to the role of parent as well as family expectations playing leading parts in the motivation to begin childbearing.

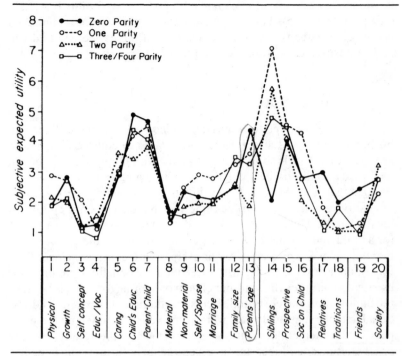

Figure 6.3 Mean Scores by Parity of Female Subjects on the 20-Level Subjective Expected Utility Scores

Once couples have a first child, they become more committed to further childbearing than they may ever be again. First-parity couples are clearly the most motivated to have another child. The most important single factor in both husbands' and wives' motivation for the second child is to provide a companion or playmate, for the first child (14: siblings). This is true both for husbands ($F = 6.99$; d.f. = 3,195; $p < .01$) and for wives ($F = 9.17$; d.f. = 3,195; $p < .01$). In fact, it remains a relatively positive motivation for childbearing at even higher parities. These data suggest that the cultural bias against the one-child family has been accepted by the couples under study.

In comparison to women at other parities, those with one child view the birth of a second child as enhancing their own maturity (3: self-concept; $F = 2.81$; d.f. = 3,195; $p < .05$) and as bringing them into a closer relationship with their husbands (10: self/spouse relationship; $F = 3.33$; d.f. = 3,195; $p < .01$). Finally, for men who already have one or more children, an incentive for continued childbearing is the positive qualities of an additional child (15: prospective child; $F = 3.20$; d.f. $= 3,195$; $p < .05$). Thus, husbands indicate that having a third child is important because the unique qualities of the expected child will have a positive impact on the family.

DISCUSSION

We have attempted to assess the subjective expected utilities that husbands and wives attach to factors related to childbearing and to see the extent to which such utilities vary with family size. To begin, we found a similarity between the way the aggregate of husbands and the aggregate of wives judge the utility of having a child. Second, a set of positive and negative utilities emerged that characterize childbearing decisions: The role of parenthood, with its opportunity for caring for a child and seeing to its education and training, and the development of a close parent-child relationship offer the principal incentives for childbearing. At each parity these positive benefits were opposed by negative utilities that another child would bring to the well-being of the family. Material costs and effects on attainment of parents' educational and occupational goals were perceived as strained by the prospect of another child. Thus, at every stage in the family-building process, further childbearing involves a set of both costs and benefits.

The results of this study suggest that decision models may provide a means of assaying and calculating the motivational basis of an individual's motivations for and against childbearing. This has practical implications for population policy, reproductive counseling, and the opportunity to try out new explanatory ideas regarding fertility at the aggregate level. The last decade has brought a more complete realization of the importance of demographic factors on social welfare. The development of programs to implement national policies would be helped by a more complete understanding of the motivational bases of childbearing. Further, improvements in contraception and the availability of legal abortion have made it increasingly possible for couples to implement their reproductive decisions. But before fertility comes within what Ansley Coale (1973) has called the "calculus of conscious choice," potential parents must consider it appropriate to balance the advantages and disadvantages of each additional birth. Unfortunately, this complex and multifaceted task requires considerably more clarity of thought and decision-making skill than most people possess. The Hierarchy provides a means of systematically assessing the factors that weigh most heavily upon individuals as they make reproductive decisions. As such, it is a useful counseling aid that has been helpful in family-planning counseling (Beach et al., 1978; Wood et al., 1977).

Of course, the study and the Hierarchy have their drawbacks. For example, we do not know how generalizable the results are; the participants in this study were primarily middle-class, fairly well educated, and predominantly white. The scoring of the Hierarchy is quite complex, as are the instructions for filling it out. This means that its use in other than a research context requires a knowledgeable person to administer and score it and to interpret the results. In a research context this is less of a problem.

To conclude, this study has demonstrated a method for returning to the old quest with a new approach. It moves away from the unproductive strategy of searching for personality and demographic characteristics that might be associated with the decision about children, and provides a method for articulating the underlying motivational bases of fertility decisions throughout the family-building process.

NOTES

1. Copies of the Hierarchy and mehods of administration and scoring may be obtained by writing to National Alliance for Optional Parenthood, 2010 Massachusetts Ave., N.W., Washington, D.C. 20036.

2. The authors wish to thank Dr. Barbara Beach for her assistance in analyzing the data.

REFERENCES

Adler, N. E. Decision models in population research. *Journal of Population*, 1979, 2, 187-202.

Beach, L. R., Campbell, F. L., and Townes, B. D. Subjective expected utility and the prediction of birth planning decisions. *Organizational Behavior and Human Performance*, 1979, 24, 18-28.

Beach, L. R., Townes, B. D., and Campbell, F. L. *The optional parenthood questionnaire.* Baltimore: National Organization for Non-Parents, 1978.

Beach, L. R., Townes, B. D., Campbell, F. L., and Keating, G. W. Developing and testing a decision aid for birth planning decisions. *Organizational Behavior and Human Performance*, 1976, 15, 99-116.

Beckman, L. J. The relative rewards and costs of parenthood and employment for employed women. *Psychology of Women Quarterly*, 1978, 2, 215-234.

Beckman, L. J., and Houser, B. B. Perceived satisfactions and costs of motherhood and employment among married women. *Journal of Population*, 1979, 2, 306-327.

Bumpass, L. L., and Westoff, C. F. The prediction of completed fertility. *Demography*, 1969, 6, 445-454.

Bumpass, L. L., and Westoff, C. F. *The later years of childbearing*. Princeton, NJ: Princeton University Press, 1970.

Coale, A. J. The demographic transition. Prepared for the International Population Conference, Liege, Belgium, 1973.

Crawford, T. J. Beliefs about birth control: A consistency theory analysis. *Representative Research in Social Psychology*, 1973, 4, 53-65.

Davidson, A. R., and Jaccard, J. J. Social-psychological determinants of fertility intentions. In S. H. Newman and V. D. Thompson (Eds.), *Population psychology: Research and educational issues*. Bethesda, MD: Department of Health, Education, and Welfare, 1976.

Easterlin, R. A. Towards a socio-economic theory of fertility: Survey of recent research on economic factors in American fertility. In *Fertility and family planning: A world view*. Ann Arbor: University of Michigan Sesquicentennial Celebration, 1967.

Fawcett, J. T. Psychological research and population policy. *Journal of Social Issues*, 1974, 30, 31-38.

Fawcett, J. T., and Arnold, F. S. The value of children: Theory and method. *Representative Research in Social Psychology*, 1973, 4, 23-35.

Freedman, R., Whelpton, P. K., and Campbell, A. A. *Family planning, sterility, and population growth*. New York: McGraw-Hill, 1959.

Goldberg, D., Sharp, H., and Freedman, R. The stability and reliability of expected family size data. *Milbank Memorial Fund Quarterly*, 1959, 37, 369-385.

Inazu, J., Langmeyer, D., and Lundgren, D. *Personal beliefs and normative beliefs about intended family size*. Paper presented at the Eighty-Second Annual Meeting of the American Psychological Association, New Orleans, August 1974.

Insko, C. A., Black, R. R., Cialdini, R. B., and Mulaik, S. A. Attitude toward birth control and cognitive consistency: Theoretical and practical implications of survey data. *Journal of Personality and Social Psychology*, 1970, 16, 228-237.

Jaccard, J. J., and Davidson, A. R. The relation of psychological, social and economic variables to fertility-related decisions. *Demography*, 1976, 13, 329-338.

Kirchner, E. P., and Seaver, W. B. *Developing measures of parenthood motivation*. Final report, Institute for Research on Human Resources, Pennsylvania State University, 1977.

Kiser, C. V. and Whelpton, P. K. Resume of the Indianapolis study of the social and psychological factors affecting fertility. *Population Studies*, 1953, 7, 95-110

Kiser, C. V., and Whelpton, P. K. Social and psychological factors affecting fertility. *Milbank Memorial Fund Quarterly*, 1958, 36, 282-329.

Kothandapani, V. Validation of feeling, belief, and intention to act as three components of attitude and their contribution to prediction of contraceptive behavior. *Journal of Personality and Social Psychology*, 1971, 19, 321-333.

Newman, S. H. and Thompson, V. D. (Eds.). *Population psychology: Research and educational issues*. Washington, DC: Government Printing Office, 1976. (017-046-00035-7)

Pohlman, E. H. *The psychology of birth planning*. Cambridge, MA: Schenkman, 1969.

Rainwater, L. *Family design: Marital sexuality, family size and contraception.* Chicago: Aldine, 1965.

Smetana, J. G., and Alder, N. E. Decision-making regarding abortion: A value X expectancy analysis. *Journal of Population,* 1979, 2, 339-357.

Townes, B. D., Beach, L. R., Campbell, F. L., and Wood, R. L. Family building: A social psychological study of fertility decisions. *Population and Environment,* 1980, 3(3/4), 210-220.

Werner, P. D., Middlestadt-Carter, S. E., and Crawford, T. J. Having a third child: Predicting behavioral intentions. *Journal of Marriage and the Family,* 1975, 37, 348-358.

Westoff, C. F., Mishler, E. G., and Kelly, E. L. Preferences in size of family and eventual fertility twenty years after. *American Journal of Sociology,* 1957, 62, 491-497.

Westoff, C. F., Potter, R. G., Jr., and Sagi, P. C. *The third child.* Princeton, NJ: Princeton University Press, 1963.

Westoff, C. F., Potter, R. G., Jr., Sagi, P. C., and Mishlev, E. G. *Family growth in metropolitan America.* Princeton, NJ: Princeton University Press, 1961.

Westoff, C. F., and Ryder, N. B. Recent trends in attitudes toward fertility control and the practice of contraception in the United States. In S. J. Behrman et al. (Eds.), *Fertility and family planning.* Ann Arbor: University of Michigan Press, 1969.

Whelpton, P. K., Campbell, A. A., and Patterson, J. E. *Fertility and family planning in the United States.* Princeton, NJ: Princeton University Press, 1966.

Whelpton, P. K., and Kiser, C. V. (Eds.), *Social and psychological factors affecting fertility in the United States.* (5 vols.). New York: Milbank Memorial Fund, 1946, 1950, 1952, 1954, 1958.

White, T. H. *The sword in the stone.* New York: Putnam, 1939.

Wood, R. J., Campbell, F. L., Townes, B. D., and Beach, L. R. Birth planning decisions. *American Journal of Public Health,* 1977, 6, 563-565.

7

Family Constellation and Parental Beliefs

Ann V. McGillicuddy-DeLisi
and Irving E. Sigel

Investigations of parents' ideal, desired, and expected family size and child spacing began several decades ago. This interest in parental preferences concerning family constellation was initially based on research questions focusing on the relationship between the type of family that individuals advocate and the actual number and spacing of children that come to form their family. It does make sense, after all, to investigate the type of family that people desire if one wishes to understand decision-making and planning regarding childbearing. Therefore, a logical place to begin was to study how similar actual outcomes in childbearing are to the ideals that prospective or new parents express concerning number and timing of births.

These early investigations of family constellation preferences were criticized, however, when a study of the relationship between such self-reports and actual number and spacing of children after a twenty-year period revealed low correlations (Westoff et al., 1957).

RESEARCH PRESENTED in this chapter was supported by Grant R01-HD10686 from the National Institutes of Health, 1976-1979.

This study suggested that what parents say they want or say is ideal in terms of a family actually bears very little resemblance to the type of family constellation that was achieved.

There are several problems, however, in assuming that parental preferences concerning the number and timing of births should be predictive of the structure of the family after a twenty-year period. It has been proposed that family size and spacing preferences might not be stable over the twenty years covered by the Westoff et al. study. For example, social standards relative to family size and the experience of having the first child might induce change in family preferences and planning (Freedman et al., 1965). This view of parents is consistent with current conceptualizations of the family as a system of mutual influence in which parents are affected by the child as well as vice versa (Bell, 1979; Lerner and Spanier, 1978; McGillicuddy-DeLisi, 1980; Hill, 1979). That is, parents' thinking about their own ability to devote time, energy, attention, and financial resources to children is likely to be affected by their experiences during the parenting years. Their view of a child's needs may alter as they obtain experience as a parent. In addition, one spouse may affect the other in terms of sharing desires and ideals concerning childbearing. In short, there are a multitude of factors within the family unit that could affect views of ideal family constellation over a twenty-year period. Thus, family size and spacing preferences most likely are not stable attributes that are predictive of family constellation after the childbearing years have ended, but rather reflect views of individuals given the current family constellation and plans for more immediate changes (a new birth as opposed to the final family constellation outcome).

The purpose of the present study was to investigate parents' views of ideal family size and child spacing, the rationales for such views, and parental views of the positive and negative effects of family constellation on the child. The aim of this research is not to predict the family constellation achieved by individuals, but rather to investigate the relationship between parental views and actual number and spacing of children currently constituting the family unit. Parents of an only child and parents of three children were selected for study based on Freedman et al.'s (1965) assumption that each birth, but especially the first birth, gives rise to couples' reviewing their preferences. Comparison of family constellation views of these two groups can provide a description of particular elements that are related to ideal and actual family size.

Currently there is little information in the literature about parents' views of ideal family constellation given the number and spacing of children forming their family units in the immediate present. In the 1970s and 1980s there have been several developments that increase the importance of investigating such views. First, with improved contraceptive methods, parents have the opportunity to exert more control over the timing of the birth of the first and subsequent children. Within the framework of the present study, this fact is not to be taken as indicating that we think the predictive power of expressed ideals to actual family constellation has increased. Rather, the likelihood that parents will *think* about optimal timing of births and consider alternatives of small versus larger family size and near versus far spacing of births is increased as a result of more control over childbearing. Second, the increase in numbers of women who wish to pursue a career and/or feel that it is necessary to continue or resume working outside of the home (see Rapoport and Rapoport, 1971) may necessitate increased consideration of optimal timing and planning of births. Finally, negative stereotypes associated with voluntary childlessness, only children, and smaller families have gradually been lessening in the United States in recent years (Falbo, 1979; Veevers, 1979). Each of these changes represents social and psychological factors that affect fertility, and each increases the likelihood that parents will consider family constellation alternatives as part of their "family design."

Given the assumption that parents do think about the timing and number of births, and that their views are dependent on the current structure of the family, we also wished to investigate whether their rationales for ideal number and spacing of children varied with the current structure of the family. For example, parents of three children might be more likely to justify their preferences on the basis of amount of parental attention available to each child, while parents of an only child might be more concerned with financial aspects of raising children. This could occur because the parent of three children has had to cope with the problem of dividing attention among the three children, while this problem has not occurred and is therefore likely to be less salient to the parent of an only child. Similarly, parents advocating close spacing between births might focus on having siblings close in age to serve as playmates for one another, while those advocating greater birth spacing might focus on the parent's energy level with respect to raising young children close in age. Thus, eliciting rationales for expressed ideals could provide information about the basis for those ideals and any variation that might occur with differences in actual number or spacing of children.

In addition, parents' views of the effects of family constellation on children's development were elicited. Prior research has indicated that parents of an only child differ from parents of three children in the way that they think children acquire some concepts and social skills (McGillicuddy-DeLisi, forthcoming). For example, parents who have one child were more likely to say that children learn through direct instruction from adults than were parents of three children. Parents with more than one child, on the other hand, believed that development was a result of the child's own activities and experiences more often than did parents of an only child. While we do not know if parents planned their families in accordance with these beliefs or if such beliefs were a result of the individual's parenting experience, there does appear to be some relationship between beliefs held by parents and the current number and spacing of children in the family. This relationship has been investigated, however, only with respect to parents' views of child development processes in general. In the present study, we specifically asked parents how they think the number, spacing, and birth order of children affects a particular child in the family. In this manner we could obtain information concerning what areas of development parents think are affected by the family constellation and investigate differences that might occur between parents of families that differ in actual number and spacing of children.

In summary, this investigation involved an intensive study of a relatively select group of families in order to obtain information about parents' views of an ideal family constellation, rationales underlying such views, and the ways in which they think the child's position in the family constellation affects that child's development. Parents of families that differed in number and spacing of children were selected in order to study differences that might occur relative to the actual family constellation at the time of the study. The research design, sample of participant families, and procedures are more fully described below.

METHOD

Sample and Design

There were 120 families residing within a fifty-mile radius of Princeton, New Jersey, who participated in the study. Volunteers were solicited through newspaper ads, public schools, library story hours, labor unions, pediatrician offices, notices in apartment-complex laundryrooms and in children's clothing and department stores. All families were paid for their participation.

Forty two-parent families with an only child aged 3½ to 4½ years old (mean 48.05 months; SD = 2.87) and 80 two-parent families with three children were selected to enable a comparison of parents' views of family constellation after the birth of several children versus after the birth of a single child. The middle child in the three-child families was also 3½ to 4½ years old (mean = 48.09 months; SD = 3.56). This age range was selected to ensure that enough time had elapsed for parents of three-child families to have experienced a birth subsequent to the target (preschool-age) child and that parents of an only child had allowed three years to elapse without experiencing another birth. Only 2 of the 40 families with an only child reported that they had desired to have another child during that period and were unable to do so for medical reasons. In order to examine the relationship between child spacing and parental family constellation views, spacing between the oldest and middle child was less than three years for 40 of the three-child families (mean = 24.70 months; SD = 5.88) and was greater than three years for 40 of the families (mean = 45.18 months; SD = 9.58).

Within each of these three family types (only child, N = 40; near spacing, N = 40; far spacing, N = 40), half of the families were characterized as working-class and half as middle-class on the basis of parental education and income levels (mean [and SD] family educational level[1] for working-class group = 12.55 [.82] years, for middle-class group = 15.78 [1.52] years; mean [and SD] family income level[2] for working-class group = 16.48 [4.62] thousands per year, middle-class group = 21.29 [4.43] thousands per year). There was an equal number of families with male and female target children in each family constellation-social class group. The oldest and middle children in the three-child families were of the same sex for 83 percent of the sample. The sex of the youngest child and spacing between the middle and youngest children were not controlled in selecting families.

An attempt was made to select families in which parents fell in a relatively narrow and young age range so that childbearing plans and decisions would be salient issues. This was true for parents with an only child and for parents of three children. As a group, mothers tended to be a few years younger than fathers. The mean (and SD) age of mothers was 29.88 (4.17), 30.50 (3.42), and 30.88 (2.99) years for families with an only child, near spacing, and far spacing, respectively. For fathers, mean (and SD) age was 32.68 (5.98), 32.12 (3.17), and 31.88 (2.75) years for each group.

Procedures

Each parent was seen individually. Questionnaires and interviews were administered at the Family Research Laboratory at Educational Testing Service. Parental views of family constellation were assessed through questionnaire and interview probes. Interviews were recorded on a cassette tape. Parents first responded to questionnaire items that required them to indicate how many children are ideal and how many years' spacing between children is ideal. In each case, parents were also asked to provide a brief statement of their reasons for considering such a family as ideal. Ideals stated for number of children and spacing were simply recorded from the questionnaire. Parental rationales for such preferences were coded as parent-oriented (for example, health of the mother, strain on marital relationship, desire to return to work), child-oriented (such as sibling to play with, amount of parental attention), or financial (what can be afforded, paying college tuition for one child at a time, and the like). Interrater agreement between two coders who scored 20 percent of the protocols independently of one another was 95 percent.

After parents completed the questionnaire they were interviewed for approximately one to two hours, responding to issues concerning optimal childrearing practices and child development processes in general. At the termination of this interview parents were asked whether they thought family size affects the child's development and how. The same questions were then asked relative to child spacing and ordinal position in the family. The effect of each family structure variable on children that was referred to by the parent was coded as positive or negative and the aspect of development (for example, cognitive, social, personality, or affective) affected was recorded. Each aspect of development was defined as follows: (1) *Cognitive:* The parent refers to an impact upon the child's intellectual functioning in general or upon particular intellectual skills, such as references to being smart or to verbal or mathematical skills. (2) *Social:* The parent describes outcomes that affect the child's relationships and interactions with other persons or the extent of socialization, such as closeness to siblings, learning rules, being outgoing or shy. (3) *Personality:* The parent refers to an aspect or the total organization of the child's distinguishing character traits, attitudes, or disposition that are relatively stable over time and situations, such as whether the child is spoiled, dependent, responsible, or confident. (4) *Affective:* The parent describes a transitory or permanent emotional state of the child that results from family constellation, such as happiness, loneliness, or feeling good. A manual describing the administration and scoring procedures in detail is available from the authors. The protocols were coded by three scorers. Interrater agreement for 20 percent of the protocols ranged from 87 to 96 percent (mean = 92 percent).

FINDINGS AND DISCUSSION

Ideal Number and Spacing of Children

The ideal number of and years of spacing between children that parents listed on the questionnaire are presented in the upper portion of Table 7.1. Chi-square tests were used to compare frequencies of cited ideals between the three family constellation groups, the two social class groups, mothers versus fathers, and parents of male versus parents of female children.

Frequencies of parents' references to ideal numbers of children were grouped as 0, 1, 2, 3, and 4 or more in order to avoid low expected cell frequencies in analyses. Chi-square tests comparing responses of mothers versus fathers and comparing parents of boys to parents of girls indicated that there were no significant differences between groups based on parent or child sex in the number of children cited as ideal. Sex of parent and of child were therefore ignored in analyses of differences that occurred with family constellation and social class, resulting in a total number of 240 responses (120 mothers and 120 fathers) in the subsequent analysis of ideal number of children.

Significant differences between the family constellation groups [χ^2 (8) = 43.69; p < .001] and between the social class groups [χ^2 (4) = 12.07; p < .05] were obtained. As Table 7.1 indicates, parents of an only child cited ideal family sizes that were smaller than those cited by parents of three-child families. Of the parents of an only child, 73 percent posited 0, 1, or 2 children as ideal, while only 40 percent of the parents of three children referred to such ideal family sizes. Note that parents of an only child responded that two children were ideal most often (58 percent) while parents of both near- and far-spacing three-child families tended to cite three children as ideal most often (40 and 43 percent, respectively). In addition, working-class parents referred

TABLE 7.1   Frequencies of Parents' Ideal Number and Spacing of Children

	Only Child				Near Spacing				Far Spacing			
	Working-Class		Middle-Class		Working-Class		Middle-Class		Working-Class		Middle-Class	
	Mother	Father	Mother	Father	Mother	Father	Mother	Father	Mother	Father	Mother	Father
Ideal number of children												
0	1	0	2	0	1	3	3	4	1	2	4	3
1	3	2	1	2	1	0	1	1	0	0	0	0
2	8	12	15	12	10	3	3	2	7	4	5	6
3	8	5	2	4	5	13	7	7	9	12	8	5
4 or more	0	1	0	2	3	1	6	6	3	2	3	6
Ideal years' spacing between children												
1	2	5	0	3	3	6	3	5	0	3	3	3
2	3	4	1	5	9	12	5	3	3	8	2	4
3	10	4	8	8	8	2	11	12	14	8	13	10
4 or more	5	7	11	4	0	0	1	0	3	1	2	3

to ideal family sizes that were larger than those cited by middle-class parents (see Table 7.1).

The number of children cited as an ideal family size was also grouped according to the relation to the actual constellation of the family. That is, each parent's response was coded as indicating an ideal that was either larger than, smaller than, or equal to the actual number of children in the family at the time of testing. As expected given the findings above, parents of an only child expressed an ideal family size larger than the actual family size more frequently than did parents in the near- and far-spacing groups (86, 20, and 18 percent, respectively; $\chi^2[4] = 101.04$; $p < .01$). Parents who had three children expressed ideals that matched their current family size more often than did parents of an only child (40, 43, and 10 percent for near-spacing, far-spacing, and only-child groups, respectively). Parents of three children were also more likely to posit an ideal family size that was smaller than their actual family than parents of an only child (40, 40, and 4 percent, respectively. Note, however, that parents of an only child necessarily posited that no children formed the ideal family size in order to conform to the definition of an ideal family size smaller than their own. Parents in families with near spacing and in families with far spacing between births responded similarly to one another with respect to ideal number of children. This raises the possibility that decisions concerning family size and child spacing may be relatively independent of one another in families with three children.

Frequencies of references to each type of rationale for the cited ideal family size are presented in Table 7.2. Parents of an only child gave fewer parent-oriented rationales and more child-oriented rationales for their smaller family size ideals than did parents of three children ($\chi^2[4] = 19.23$; $p < .01$). Parents of an only child also cited financial reasons for such ideals more often than did other parents.

Ideal number of years' spacing between children varied with family constellation ($\chi^2[6] = 39.17$; $p < .001$) and with sex of parent ($\chi^2[3] = 9.93$; $p < .05$). As indicated in the lower portion of Table 7.1, parents of an only child cited four or more years' spacing as ideal more often than did parents of three children (34 versus 1 and 11 percent for near- and far-spacing groups). Parents with near spacing referred to one or two years' spacing as ideal more often than did other parents. In addition, mothers tended to cite greater spacing as ideal more

TABLE 7.2   Reference to Each Type of Rationale for Ideal Number and Spacing of Children

Type of Rationale	Family Constellation (percentages)		
	Only Child	Near Spacing	Far Spacing
Ideal size			
Parent	21	47	44
Child	46	28	39
Financial	33	24	17
Ideal spacing			
Parent	27	32	46
Child	72	67	54
Financial	1	1	1

frequently than fathers. For example, 53 percent of the mothers referred to three years' spacing as ideal, while only 37 percent of the fathers cited three years as ideal.

Frequencies of parents whose ideals deviated or matched current child spacing were not analyzed, since none of the parents of an only child and none of the parents with far child spacing indicated an ideal spacing that exceeded the spacing of their own family. Inspection of the data for near-spaced families did reveal that 39 percent of these parents (total possible = 80) expressed an ideal spacing that was greater than that evidenced in their own families. Ideal child spacing matched actual child spacing for 41 near-spacing, 44 far-spacing, and 27 only-child parents, where a match was defined as age of the target plus one year for parents of an only child. Ideal spacing was less than actual child spacing for 0 near-spacing, 26 far-spacing, and 53 only-child family parents. Rationales for ideal spacing also varied with family constellation, as indicated in Table 7.2 (χ^2 [2] = 9.81; p < .01, omitting financial category to achieve required cell frequencies). Most parents referred to child-oriented reasons for ideal spacing, regardless of the actual family constellation, but parents with far spacing between children did cite parent-oriented rationale more frequently than did other parents.

To summarize thus far, parental views of ideal family size tended to be consistent with the actual family constellation for the most part. The exception was the case of parents of an only child, who cited an ideal family size of two children most often (59 percent). These parents also indicated that three or four years' spacing between children was ideal, suggesting that these one-child families may have been incomplete at the time of testing. However, a follow-up questionnaire two years after testing showed that only 13 of the 40 one-child families had experienced the birth of a second child. This raises the question of whether the parents were hesitant to cite one child as ideal, indicating that negative stereotypes associated with the only child may still exist and social desirability factors mitigated parental responses. Ten percent of the parents expressed an ideal family size that included no children, and it was somewhat surprising that this was slightly more frequent in three-child families than in one-child families (26 versus 8 percent). This finding might be due to the increasing acceptance of stating that one does not desire to be a parent, or may indicate a reaction to the stress of being a parent in a larger family by today's standard of family size (see Bell et al., 1980).

Ideal spacing also tended to reflect the spacing evidenced in the actual family constellation, although not to the same degree as was evidenced with number of children. Nearly 33 percent of the parents with far spacing between children expressed an ideal spacing that was less than that evidenced in their own families, and 49 percent of the parents with near-spaced families ideally preferred greater spacing between children. It is likely that this reflects the greater control of parents over number of children as opposed to timing of births subsequent to the first child.

Views of Effects of Family Constellation

The number of references to positive and negative effects of family size, child spacing, and birth order on the child are presented in percentages in Table 7.3 by family constellation group. A $3 \times 2 \times 2 \times 2$ (family constellation x social class x parent sex x child sex) analysis of variance indicated significant effects between the family constellation groups for (1) positive effects of a large family ($F [2/119] = 5.43$; $p < .01$); (2) positive effects of far spacing ($F [2/119] = 3.83$; $p < .02$); (3) negative effects of far spacing ($F [2/119] = 4.89$; $p < .01$); (4) negative effects of being firstborn ($F [2/119] = 4.42$; $p < .01$); (5) positive effects of being a middle child ($F [2/119] = 10.24$; $p < .001$); (6) negative effects of being last born ($F [2/119] = 5.55$; $p < .01$); and (7) negative effects of being an only child ($F [2/119] = 5.55$; $p < .01$). In addition, effects for sex of parent were obtained for (1) negative effects of a large family ($F [1/119] = 3.86$; $p < .05$); (2) negative effects of near spacing ($F [1/119] = 3.74$; $p < .05$); and (3) negative effects of being middle

TABLE 7.3   References to Positive and Negative Effects of Family
Constellation on a Child's Development

	Family Constellation Groups (percentages)		
	Only Child	Near Spacing	Far Spacing
Family size[a]			
Large+	46	61	85
Large−	78	59	60
Small+	41	41	51
Small−	10	19	19
Spacing			
Far+	43	18	29
Far−	53	84	79
Near+	48	73	54
Near−	58	36	65
Birth order			
First+	58	49	58
First−	36	54	68
Middle+	11	26	50
Middle−	48	58	53
Last+	31	29	41
Last−	33	43	64
Only+	33	20	33
Only−	48	91	100

a. (+) denotes a positive effect and (−) a negative effect.

born ($F[1/119] = 9.56$; $p < .01$). Also, an SES effect was obtained for
negative effects of far spacing ($F[1/119] = 6.79$; $p < .01$).

In general, Scheffé tests indicated that parental views of positive
and negative effects of family constellation were concordant with the
actual family structure. Parents with three children in both spacing
groups referred to positive aspects of growing up in a large family
more often than did parents of an only child. With regard to spacing,
parents of an only child referred to positive aspects of far spacing
more often and to negative aspects of near spacing less often than did
parents with three children. With regard to birth order, parents of an
only child referred to negative aspects of being both a firstborn child
and being an only child less frequently than did parents with three
children. Parents with far spacing between children were different
from parents with near spacing and from parents with an only child in
their views about middle and youngest children. Positive aspects of
being a middle child and negative aspects of being a last born were

expressed more often by parents in the far-spacing group than by parents in the other two groups.

With respect to differences between mothers and fathers, 75 percent of the fathers cited negative consequences of a large family on the child, as opposed to only 57 percent of the mothers. Mothers, on the other hand, cited negative effects more often than did fathers for near spacing (67 and 40 percent, respectively) and for being a middle child (67 and 38 percent, respectively). The social class effect for negative effects of far spacing was due to higher frequency of such a view among working-class parents (84 percent) than among middle-class parents (60 percent).

Areas of child development that parents viewed as affected by family constellation also varied with the actual structure of the family. The number of parental references to positive and negative effects on cognitive, social, personality, and affective development are presented in Table 7.4. Analyses of variance yielded significant effects between family constellation groups for number of references to (1) negative effects on social development ($F[2/119] = 3.58$; $p < .05$); (2) positive effects on personality development ($F[2/119] = 4.42$; $p < .01$); and (3) negative effects on personality development ($F[2/119] = 7.74$; $p < .001$). Significant main effects for social class occurred for (1) positive effects on personality development ($F[1/119] = 7.06$; $p < .001$) and (2) positive effects on affective development ($F[1/119] = 4.92$; $p < .05$). In addition, a family constellation × social class interaction was obtained for positive effects on personality development ($F[2/119] = 3.53$; $p < .05$).

Parents of an only child expressed the view that the structure of the family could negatively affect both personality and social development less often than did parents of three children. Parents of families with far spacing between children referred to positive effects of family constellation on a child's personality more often than did parents with near spacing between children or parents of an only child. Middle-class parents referred to positive effects of family constellation on both personality and affective development more often than did working-class parents. Middle-class parents with far spacing between children referred to positive effects of family constellation on children's personality more often than did parents in all other groups.

In summary, references to positive and negative effects of family constellation on the child varied with actual family constellation and to some extent with the sex of the parent and social class. Parents'

TABLE 7.4   References to Areas of the Child's Development That Are Affected by Family Constellation

| Area of Development[a] | Family Constellation and Social Class Groups (percentages) | | | | | |
| | Only Child | | Near Spacing | | Far Spacing | |
	Working-class	Middle-class	Working-class	Middle-class	Working-class	Middle-class
Cognitive+	20	11	13	15	18	18
Cognitive−	7	6	2	7	4	5
Social+	45	36	41	47	46	64
Social−	32	23	42	32	45	42
Personality+	14	22	18	17	18	42
Personality−	25	18	38	35	39	47
Emotional+	9	13	7	13	8	17
Emotional−	29	20	36	17	35	25

a. (+) denotes a positive effect and (−) a negative effect.

views of the positive and negative effects of family size and spacing were consistent with the number and spacing of children in their families, for the most part. Parents with three children cited positive effects of large families, negative effects of far spacing, and only-child status more often than did parents of one child. Although there were no differences between family constellation groups, references to negative effects of a small family were minimal. Fathers and mothers differed from one another with respect to views on effects of a large family, near spacing, and being a middle child. In addition, working-class parents saw negative effects of far spacing on the child more often than did middle-class parents.

With respect to effects of birth order on children's development, it was somewhat surprising that only about half of the parents referred to negative effects of being a middle child and that firstborn and/or last-born status was seen as carrying as much negative effect as the middle position in the family. Parents of an only child were, however, less likely than other parents to cite negative aspects of being a firstborn and less likely than parents with far spacing between children to cite negative effects of being last born.

Most parents focused on social and personality development when they were asked if and what aspects of a child's development were affected by family constellation: 81 percent of the parents did not think that cognitive development of children was affected by family constellation, either positively or negatively. This indicates that references to decrements in IQ with increased family size in the popular literature have not had much impact on parents' views of the relationship between family size and children's intellectual ability. Parents of three children were more likely to posit family constellation effects on children's personality and affective development than were parents of an only child, and both social class and child spacing were related to parents' views of the positive effects of family constellation on children's personality development.

SUMMARY AND CONCLUSIONS

In general, parental views of ideal family size and child spacing varied with actual number and spacing of children in the family. In addition, parental views of the effects of family constellation on the child's development varied with actual family constellation in such a manner that it appears that actual family structure reflects parental views of what is best for the child. While the design of the present study does not enable investigation of the question of whether parents planned their families in accordance with such views or if such views have been affected by the particular constellation that exists, it is clear that parents of an only child view family constellation effects quite differently than do parents of three children.

The types of rationales given for views of ideal number of children and the results pertaining to views of effects of family constellation indicate that most parents of an only child feel that large families do not have a positive effect on the child and that their ideals of smaller families are based on what is best for the child. Parents of an only child do not view family constellation as having a negative effect on children's social and personality development as often as do parents of three children, and the references to effects of birth order on the child are less frequent than for parents of three children. Regardless of whether such views existed prior to parenthood or not, it appears that family size is related to the parents' conception of the ways in which family constellation affect the child.

Results pertaining to the relationship between family constellation and child development beliefs in general provide further support for the notion that the actual family constellation is related to the parents' views of what is best for the child. It has been reported elsewhere that parents of an only child refer to adult instruction and guidance as the processes through which children learn concepts and gain knowledge more than do parents of three children. Parents of three children, on the other hand, refer to peer influence, self-regulation, and observation more often than do parents of one child (see McGillicuddy-DeLisi, forthcoming). Results of the present study suggest that parents of an only child and parents of three children may also differ from one another in their views of what affects the personal-social development of the child. That is, parents of three children referred to effects of family constellation on this area of development more often than did parents of an only child.

Effects indicating differences between mothers and fathers raise some important issues regarding decision-making and childbearing. Mothers generally preferred greater spacing between births and viewed near spacing and the middle-birth position as having negative consequences for the child more often than did fathers. Mothers were also less likely to cite negative consequences of a large family on the child than fathers were. These results raise the question of how such discrepancies, if they occur within a particular family, are resolved between husband and wife. They also suggest that mothers may be more exposed to "expert advice," in that greater spacing is currently being advocated in the popular and professional literature.

In conclusion, parental views of family constellation appear to be linked to the actual number and spacing of children in the family. Whether parents plan their families in accordance with such views or justify their own family unit after the fact, it is likely that decisions regarding the family design are influenced by the parents' view of how the family unit affects the child. Regardless of how many children parents have, or the spacing between them, parents tend to express the view that their own particular family constellation matches an ideal of what is best for children, and this focus is relative to the personal-social development of the child rather than upon cognitive development fostered in the family environment.

NOTES

1. Family educational level = (number of years of formal schooling for father + number of years of formal schooling for mother)/2.
2. Family income level = father's yearly income plus mother's yearly income at time of testing.

REFERENCES

Bell, C. S., Johnson, J. E., McGillicuddy-DeLisi, A. V., and Sigel, I. E. Normative stress and young families: Adaptation and development. *Family Relations,* 1980, 29, 453-458.

Bell, R. Parent, child and reciprocal influences. *American Psychologist,* 1979, 34, 821-826.

Falbo, T. The only child: A review. In G. K. Phelan (Ed.), *Family relationships.* Minneapolis: Burgess, 1979.

Freedman, R., Coombs, L. C., and Bumpass, L. Stability and change in expectations about family size: A longitudinal study. *Demography,* 1965, 2, 250-275.

Hill, R. *Theories and research designs linking family behavior and child development: A critical overview.* Paper presented at the Sixteenth International Family Research Seminar on the Child and the Family, St. Peter, Minnesota, August 1979.

Lerner, R. M., and Spanier, G. B. *Child influences on marital and family interaction.* New York: Academic Press, 1978.

McGillicuddy-DeLisi, A. V. The role of parental beliefs in the family as a system of mutual influences. *Family Relations,* 1980, 29, 317-323.

McGillicuddy-DeLisi, A. V. The relation between family configuration and parental beliefs about child development. In L. Laosa and I. E. Sigel (Eds.), *Families as learning environments for children.* New York: Plenum, forthcoming.

Rapoport, R., and Rapoport, R. N. *Dual career families.* Harmondsworth, England: Penguin, 1971.

Veevers, J. E. Voluntarily childless wives: An exploratory study. In G. K. Phelan (Ed.), *Family relationships.* Minneapolis: Burgess, 1979.

Westoff, C. F., Mishler, E. G., and Kelly, E. L. Preferences in size of family and eventual fertility twenty years after. *American Journal of Sociology,* 1957, 62, 491-497.

8

Early Mother-Child Interaction

FAMILIES WITH ONLY AND FIRSTBORN CHILDREN

Candice Feiring and Michael Lewis

The need for family-planning information has risen in recent years as the decision to have only one as opposed to more than one child has become salient. On one hand, growing concern about the consequences of overpopulation, in addition to personal economic concerns, creates pressure to produce fewer children. On the other hand, the persistent negative stereotypes concerning only children create pressure to produce more than one child. A central theme in the recent work on only children has been the importance of avoiding the negative stereotyped notions that only children are characterized by selfishness, loneliness, or maladjustment (Falbo, 1977; Thompson, 1974). Pinner and Thompson (1974) found that the concept of only children was rated more negatively on semantic

PREPARATION OF this chapter was supported by Grant NO1-HD-82849 from the Center for Population Research of the National Institute of Child Health and Human Development.

differentials and on the adjective checklist (Gough, 1952) than was the concept of a child with two siblings. Although recently there has been a growing research commitment to clarify family-planning issues, precise answers that can be tailored to the needs of individual families are not yet available. Examples of the great variety of questions to which couples are likely to want answers include (1) Can being an only child be harmful to the child's social acceptability or mental health? (2) Are only children more "spoiled" than children with siblings? (3) Do parents who have only one child become overprotective or too dependent on the child? (4) Is it inevitable that a firstborn child will suffer feelings of rejection when a sibling is born?

Research in psychology relevant to family-planning issues is most obvious in the literature on the effects of birth order. The greatest impetus to the systematic study of birth-order effects was provided by Schachter (1959), who observed that under anxiety-provoking conditions, firstborn female subjects were more likely to seek out the company of others than were later-born females. Schachter suggested that through the initial experience as the sole focus of parental love and attention, the firstborn comes to associate the reduction of its needs with the presence of others. Later-born children do not enjoy the experience of being the exclusive focus of attention and thus have to acquire strategies for need reduction through their own efforts. Schachter argued that in later life firstborns manifest greater affiliative dependence on others and conform more to the influence of others than do later-born children.

Since Schachter's original publication, research on the effects of family constellation has been characterized by the failure to examine only children separately from firstborns with younger siblings (see Greenberg, 1967; Hoyt and Raven, 1973; Toman and Toman, 1970) and the use primarily of adult subjects. In a paper on social issues involving family size, Thompson (1974) effectively argued that if family size recommendations are going to reflect a greater understanding of the psychological outcomes for children, adults, and society of having one or more children, a greater research effort is needed which distinguishes the behavioral outcomes for only children from those for children with siblings. Thompson suggests that since firstborns experience many events (in particular, "dethroning") that only children do not, it is likely that these groups differ in behavioral patterns.

In fact, firstborns and only children are probably similar only in widely spaced families. The importance of examining more closely the early experiences of firstborn children is suggested by Dunn's (1979) recent research on families with young siblings. In the context of family relationships, the changes in firstborns after the birth of a sibling, the role of the new sibling in the social development of the firstborn, and the social and cognitive development of the new sibling were examined. This research indicated that the interactions between a firstborn child and a new sibling as young as 8 months are complex, varied, and different from the interactions that children have with their parents.

The view that only children and children with siblings need to be studied separately is also supported by Eiduson's (1976) paper on the dynamics unique to the one-child family. Eiduson believes that the most salient feature distinguishing the only child's socialization is that there is only one child to absorb parental interest and attention, a situation that results in the only child becoming like his or her parents in behavior and interests, the playing of multiple roles by the parents (as playmate and/or confidant as well as caregiver), and early adultlike adjustment for the child. The importance of parents for only children has been demonstrated by Gewirtz and Gewirtz (1965), who found that mothers of only children interacted with their children twice as much as did mothers of last borns.

Although the recent and growing research effort in the areas of birth order and family constellation has addressed some issues relevant to family planning with respect to older children and adults (see Falbo, forthcoming; Thompson, 1974; Zajonc, 1976), there is little empirical information regarding the early differences between children with and without siblings. Since a clearer understanding of the source of these differences can emerge through close observation of the very young in interaction with the mother, this study emphasized the cognitive and social development of firstborn and only children within the context of the mother-child relationship. It was hoped that such an approach would provide a more precise understanding of whether and how differences in development emerge for children with and without siblings. More specifically, the focus of this study was on the differences and similarities in the social and cognitive development of firstborn and only children as observed at 3, 12, and 24 months of age.

METHOD

Defining the Sample

Fifty-six firstborn children were observed at 3, 12, and 24 months of age. The sample consisted of 21 only children (children who did not acquire a sibling in the first 48 months of life) and 35 firstborn children (children who acquired a sibling between the ages of 24 and 36 months). Of the 21 only children, 12 were female and 9 were male. Of the 35 firstborn children, 16 were female and 19 were male. It should be noted that all the analyses comparing only and firstborn children at 3 and 12 months were retrospective in nature. That is, in reality, all children were only borns, that is, had no siblings at 3 and 12 months of age. By 24 months of age, 10 children had actually become firstborns while the remainder of the sample of firstborns acquired siblings by (or soon after) 36 months of age.

Observation and Recording of Mother-Infant
Interaction at Age 3 Months:
Home Observation

Each mother-infant pair was observed in the home for a two-hour period while the infant was awake. Preparatory to observation, the observer briefly explained the purpose of the observation, showed the mother the materials being used, tried to put the mother at ease, and instructed the mother to continue with her normal routine and to ignore the observer. Upon completion of the two hours of observation, mothers were given a general-information questionnaire concerning the child's history, parental demographic characteristics, and issues pertaining to childbirth and family planning.

Infant behaviors coded at 3 months were (1) eyes closed, (2) vocalization, (3) extra movement, (4) fret/cry, (5) feed-bottle, (6) feed-spoon, (7) play-object, (8) play-person, (9) play-self, (10) smile/laugh, (11) burp, sneeze, cough, (12) looking at mother, and (13) sucking-nonfeed. Mother behaviors coded at 3 months were (1) touch, (2) hold, (3) vocalization, (4) vocalization to other, (5) look, (6) smile/laugh, (7) play with child, (8) change diaper/bathe, (9) feed, (10) rock child, (11) read/TV, (12) kiss, and (13) give toy/pacifier.

All behaviors (13 for the mother and 13 for the infant) were coded every 10 seconds on machine-scorable checklists; primary activities (such as crib or lap) were noted for each one-minute interval. In order to ensure accurate timing for coding behavior, the observer used a small timing device that only she could hear. At 3 months, behaviors were coded in ten-second intervals; the frequency data presented here reflect the number of ten-second intervals in which the behavior occurred for two hours of home observation.

Observation and Recording of Mother-Infant Interactions at Ages 12 and 24 Months: Playroom Observation

At ages 12 and 24 months, mother-infant dyads were observed in a playroom at the laboratory. The dyad was left alone in the 10x12 foot playroom, which was marked with carpet squares and contained 13 toys, a chair, a table, and a magazine. Both mother and infant were observed through a one-way mirror and videotaped. The observation consisted of a fifteen-minute free-play period in an unstructured situation in which mother and infant had the opportunity to interact with toys.

While watching the mother-child dyad through a one-way mirror, an observer dictated the ongoing behaviors and interactions onto tape so that these behaviors could later be transcribed and coded onto machine-readable sheets for analysis. Each sheet represented fifteen seconds of time; thus the fifteen-minute free-play period consisted of 60 fifteen-second periods of observation. At 12 and 24 months the frequency data presented here reflect the number of fifteen-second intervals in which a behavior occurred over 60 such fifteen-second intervals of fifteen minutes of mother-child observation.

Infant behaviors coded at 12 and 24 months were (1) vocalization, (2) looking, (3) smile, (4) touch, (5) fret/cry, (6) seek approval, (7) seek help, (8) gesture, (9) seek proximity, (10) toy/nontoy, (11) move/door, (12) lap, and (13) hold/hug. Maternal behaviors coded at 12 and 24 months were (1) vocalization, (2) looking, (3) smile, (4) touch, (5) kiss, (6) hold, (7) give directions, (8) read, (9) seek proximity, (10) toy/ nontoy, (11) show toy, (12) manipulate toy, and (13) demonstrate toy. At 12 and 24 months, for analysis purposes, mother behaviors were grouped as proximal (such as touch, kiss, hold, proximity) and distal (such as vocalize, look, smile, give directions). Infant behaviors were also grouped as proximal (such as same square, touch, seek proximity, lap, hold/hug) and distal (such as vocalize, look, smile, fret/cry, gesture).

Cognitive Assessment of Firstborn and
Only Children at 3, 12, and 24 Months

At each measurement point, the children's cognitive performance was tested using the Bayley Mental Scale of Infant Development (MDI). At 3 months of age, MDI items 26 through 73 were administered to the infants during the home visit. These items represent an average age placement from 2.1 to 5.8 months, according to Bayley. At 12 and 24 months, the MDI was administered to the children on a visit to the Infant Laboratory. This visit was made on an occasion separate from the one made for observation of mother-child interaction (the order of visits for social and cognitive testing were randomized across subjects). At 12 months of age children were given items 99 through 125 of the MDI, which represent an average age placement ranging from 11.3 to 17.8 months, according to Bayley. At 24 months of age children were administered items 124 through 163, which represent an age placement range from 17.8 months to 30+ months. It should be noted that at 3, 12, and 24 months additional measures of cognitive performance were adminstered to the sample. However, since these measures were not given at each age point and because they did not yield significant differences between firstborn and only children, they are not considered in this report.

RESULTS

Means were generated for the social behavior of infants and mothers at each age point, with the sample divided according to first and only categories. Because the data were not normally distributed, the Mann-Whitney U test was used for comparison between groups. The results are presented by the three age levels (3, 12, and 24 months) at which assessment occurred, with infant data followed by the mother data within each age level.

Age 3 Months

Infant Behavior. The upper portion of Table 8.1 presents the infant's social and cognitive behavior at 3 months of age for the total sample as well as for first and only groups. The social data in Table 8.1 are the mean numbers of ten-second intervals during which an infant behavior occurred at least once during two hours of home observation. The infant social data at 3 months suggest that firstborn children

TABLE 8.1   Infant and Maternal Behavior at 3 Months[a]

	Total N = 56	Only N = 21	First N = 35
Infant			
Close eyes	6.59	7.24	6.20
Voc	163.2	158.0	166.4
Extra movement	92.5	97.4	89.5
Cry	70.8	83.5	63.2
Feed/bottle	91.4	90.3	92.1
Feed/spoon	22.7	19.5	24.6
Play/object	138.7	132.4	142.4
Play/person	15.7	13.4	17.1
Play/self	15.3	11.0	18.0
Smile	47.5	34.5	55.2
Burp/sneeze	19.0	22.2	17.1
Look	160.5	157.5	162.3
Suck	59.9	50.5	65.5
Bayley MDI[b]	100.0	98.22	101.07
Mother			
Touch	85.0	98.6	76.9
Hold	230.0	228.1	231.1
Voc	260.3	276.1	250.9
Voc/other	127.6	146.1	116.6
Look	312.9	330.3	302.5
Smile	96.3	98.0	95.3
Play	41.5	49.7	36.6
Bathe	59.5	65.2	56.1
Feed	114.9	106.8	119.8
Rock	28.8	51.1	15.6
Read/TV	26.3	32.1	22.8
Kiss	13.9	20.2	10.1
Toy	24.0	24.8	23.7

a. The social data present the mean number of 10-second intervals that a behavior occured at least once in the two-hour observation in the home

b. Note that performance scores on the Bayley have been converted to standard scores (Mean = 100, S = 15), since only portions of the MDI were administered and not the entire scale.

are less fussy and more sociable than those children who will remain only borns (at least for the opening 48 months of life). More specifically, firstborns show a tendency to play, smile, vocalize, suck and feed by spoon more frequently than do only borns. These differences are significant for feed by spoon (Mann-Whitney U Test: $p < .05$) and almost significant for smile Mann-Whitney U Test: p < .10). Only-born infants show a tendency to cry, move, and burp/sneeze more frequently than do firstborns, with crying approaching a significant difference (Mann-Whitney U Test: p ≤ .10).

At 3 months of age, firstborn and only children do not differ significantly on the Bayley test of cognitive performance, although firstborns show a tendency to score slightly higher than only borns.

Mother Behavior. The lower portion of Table 8.1 presents the mother's social behavior when her infant was 3 months of age for the total sample as well as for first and only groups. The mother's social data, reported in Table 8.1, give the mean number of ten-second intervals during which a behavior occurred at least once during two hours of home observation. When their infants are 3 months of age, mothers of onlies more frequently rock (Mann-Whitney U Test: p < .01) and kiss (Mann-Whitney U Test: p < .05) their children as compared to mothers of firstborns. Although the differences are not significant, mothers of onlies show a tendency to touch, play, look, vocalize, and engage in more proximal and distal contact with their infants, as compared to mothers of firstborns. Feeding is the only proximal contact behavior that mothers of firsts perform more (but not significantly more) than mothers of onlies. While mothers of onlies are more frequently involved with their infants, they also are more frequently involved in noninfant-focused activities. More specifically, mothers of onlies show a tendency (a nonsignificant trend) to vocalize more frequently to persons other than the infant and to read and/or watch television, as compared to mothers of firstborns.

Maternal Interview Data: Parental Characteristics and Attitudes Toward Childbirth and Planning. Although we chose to select and examine our sample in terms of a distinction related to the child's status in regard to siblings, an equal concern in our analysis was the maternal behavior that is related to the child's development. Since the parents of only and firstborn children were an essential component of our study, it was important to determine some relevant demographic characteristics and family-planning attitudes of the mothers in our sample. From the interviews of the mothers when their children were 3 months of age, we gathered data on the mothers such as the following: occupation, education, age at child's birth, normalcy of pregnancy and delivery, attitude toward the pregnancy, and ideal family size.

TABLE 8.2   Child Behavior Frequencies at 12 and 24 Months

	12 Months			24 Months		
	Total N = 53	Only N = 21	Firsts N = 32	Total N = 49	Only N = 18	Firsts N = 31
Voc	20.3	18.0	21.7	37.4	35.8	38.4
Look	13.1	11.2	14.3	18.7	18.8	18.7
Smile	6.0	7.1	5.2	9.2	9.0	9.4
Touch	1.2	1.3	1.2	.6	.6	.7
Cry	.6	.2	.8	.8	.1	1.2
Seek approval	.02	.0	.0	.2	.0	.3
Seek help	.1	.14	.0	.8	.4	.9
Gesture	1.2	1.5	1.1	3.5	2.8	3.9
Seek proximity	.6	.3	.8	.5	.5	.55
Toy play	50.0	50.9	49.5	52.2	53.4	51.5
Move door	.1	.14	.1	.9	.4	1.2
Lap	.1	.3	.0	.8	.1	1.2
Hug	.0	.0	.0	.04	.1	.0
Proximal	11.9	13.5	10.9	17.1	14.9	18.3
Distal	41.1	38.0	43.1	69.7	66.5	71.6
Total social	93.8	91.8	95.2	158.0	125.4	129.5
Bayley MDI[a]	100.00	95.10	102.97	100.00	98.79	100.63

a. Note that performance scores on the Bayley have been converted to standard scores (Mean = 100, S = 15), since only portions of the MDI were administered and not the entire scale.

Analyses of the data from the interviews of the mothers when their first children were 3 months of age suggest that mothers of firstborn children reported a significantly higher ideal family size compared to mothers of onlies (2.75 for firsts versus 2.16 for onlies, t (48) = 2.66; p ≤ .01) and tended to feel better about becoming pregnant (94 versus 76 percent were happy or very happy for the mothers of firsts and onlies, respectively). For the mothers of firstborns, 89 percent of the pregnancies and deliveries were normal, whereas this percentage is slightly less for mothers of onlies (71 percent). Mothers of onlies tended to be slightly older at the birth of the first child than mothers of firsts ($\overline{X} = 27.9$ and $\overline{X} = 26.3$ for mothers of onlies and firsts, respectively; t (50) = 1.65; p ≤ .10). In summary, mothers of firstborns tend to be younger at the birth of the first child, express the desire for more children, and indicate a more positive attitude toward their becoming and being pregnant and delivering, as opposed to mothers of onlies.

Age 12 Months

Infant Behavior. Table 8.2 presents the infant's social and cognitive behavior at 12 months (left side) and 24 months (right side) for the total sample and by first and only groups. The social data in Table 8.2 report the mean number of fifteen-second intervals during which an infant behavior occurred at least once during fifteen minutes of free-play observation in the laboratory setting. At 12 months of age there is a nonsignificant tendency for firstborn children to show more distal and less proximal modes of contact with mother, as compared to only-born children. Otherwise, firstborn and only children are strikingly similar on all social behaviors observed at 12 months of age in the infant-mother interaction. In regard to cognitive performance, firstborn children score higher on the Bayley MDI compared to only-born children (Mann-Whitney U Test: $p < .02$), although the actual difference in mean score is a small one.

Mother Behavior. Table 8.3 presents the mother's social behavior at 12-month (left side) and 24-month (right side) assessment levels for the total sample and by first and only groups. The mother's social data, reported in Table 8.3, show the mean number of fifteen-second periods during which a behavior occurred at least once during fifteen minutes of free-play observation in the laboratory. Although the mean differences are small, mothers of onlies compared to firsts more frequently touch (Mann-Whitney U Test: $p < .001$), engage in proximal contact (Mann-Whitney U Test: $p < .01$), and play with (Mann-Whitney U Test: $p \leq .05$) their children. Mothers of firsts show a nonsignificant tendency to use the distal mode of interaction and read more frequently than do mothers of onlies. In regard to other behaviors, such as vocalization, look, smile, and give directions, mothers of firsts and onlies were very similar.

Age 24 Months

Infant Behavior. As examination of Table 8.2 indicates, firstborn and only children are very similar on all social behaviors observed at 24 months. Although firstborns show slightly more frequent use of proximal and distal modes of contact than only borns, these differences are small and not reliable.

At 24 months, the two groups of firstborn and only children do not differ significantly on the Bayley MDI. However, at this point it should be recalled that at 3 and 12 months all analyses comparing only

TABLE 8.3 Maternal Behavior Frequencies at 12 and 24 Months

	12 Months			24 Months		
	Total N=53	Only N=21	Firsts N=32	Total N=49	Only N=18	Firsts N=31
Voc	29.5	28.8	30.0	44.4	44.1	44.6
Look	48.4	48.0	48.6	45.1	44.9	45.3
Smile	21.0	19.8	21.8	16.6	14.2	18.0
Touch	2.1	3.0	1.5	2.4	2.5	2.4
Kiss	.04	.05	.0	.1	.2	.1
Hold	.3	.4	.2	.4	.3	.5
Give directions	3.0	2.8	3.2	4.9	5.0	4.8
Read	7.8	4.8	9.7	6.1	8.4	4.8
Maintain proximity	.0	.0	.0	.0	.0	.0
Toy play	13.6	17.0	11.3	16.7	17.6	16.2
Show approval	1.0	1.0	.9	3.0	3.6	2.7
Proximal	2.4	3.4	1.8	2.9	3.0	2.9
Distal	109.7	104.1	113.3	114.0	111.8	115.3
Total	127.0	126.1	127.7	141.4	142.5	140.7

borns and firstborns were retrospective in nature, while by 24 months ten children had actually become firstborns. Although the number of children who had acquired a sibling by 2 years of age is small, results pertaining to how changes in cognitive performance are related to the birth of a second sibling are of sufficient theoretical and practical interest to merit examination. Although the results are apparently clear for cognitive performance, they must be interpreted cautiously in light of the univen distribution and small sample sizes. At 24 months, those firstborn children who had acquired a sibling between 12 and 24 months performed significantly lower (Mann-Whitney U Test: $p < .05$) on the Bayley ($\overline{X}$ = 93.06), as compared to firstborns who had not yet acquired a sibling ($\overline{X}$ = 100.83) or only borns ($\overline{X}$ = 98.79). This finding is of particular note in contrast to the 12-months data, which indicated that firstborns who were to acquire a sibling between 12 and 24 months scored the highest on the Bayley MDI ($\overline{X}$ = 105.63), as compared to firstborns who would acquire a sibling after 24 months ($\overline{X}$ = 102.97) or only borns ($\overline{X}$ = 95.10). These data suggest that the birth and presence of a second child affects the firstborn child, and this may be a source of difference between first and only-born children.

Mother Behavior. Examination of the data presented in the right side of Table 8.3 indicates that, in general, mothers of first and only-born children are very similar in their social behavior as observed in the laboratory at 24 months. Although mothers of firstborns show a tendency to smile more frequently, use the distal mode of contact, and read less as compared to mothers of onlies, these differences are small and insignificant. While mothers of onlies display a tendency (Mann-Whitney U test: p < .10) to show more approval than mothers of firsts, the mean difference between groups in this behavior is very small.

DISCUSSION

The study presented here constitutes one of the few research efforts that provides empirical, longitudinal information on the behavior of first and only-born children and their mothers at early age points. Although the small sample size necessitates cautious interpretation of the data, examination of the results on the social and cognitive behavior of firstborn and only children and their mothers suggest that observed differences in these groups could be due to several sources of variation. In particular, the findings indicate that differences in only and firstborn groups could be due to (1) differences in the characteristics and behavior of the child, (2) differences in the characteristics and behavior of the parent, and (3) the birth and presence of a second child. Although we realize that these three sources of variation are not independent of each other and do not necessarily cover all possible sources of differences, we shall discuss our findings as they pertain to these three sources of variation.

As we focus our discussion on the differences in the only and firstborn groups, we must remind the reader that the observed differences, although reliable, were often quite small. Furthermore, we wish to emphasize that at each age point firstborn and only groups were very similar on several of the measures, especially at the later age point.

Differences in Firstborn and Only-Born Children
Related to Child Characteristics

The first possible source for differences in only and firstborn children concerns the characteristics of the children themselves. Firstborn and only children may be different due to variations in temperament, personality, or cognitive factors. The model of the passive child who is socialized by responding to its environment, in particular the young child responding to its parents, has been fairly well refuted (see Bell, 1971; Lewis and Rosenblum, 1974). The effect of the child on the parent-child interactions has been observed to vary with such factors as sex of child (Lewis, 1972; Parke and Sawin, 1975), age of child (Harper, 1975), and child temperament (Carey, 1970; Chess et al., 1976; Feiring, 1975). Thus, it may certainly be the case that children who will remain onlies as compared to children who will acquire a sibling may be different in ways that influence their parents' decisions concerning family planning and whether or when to have more children.

The data presented here suggest that at 3 months of age only and firstborn children are different, even though neither group has acquired a sibling (that is, even though in reality they are all only children). Only children show a tendency to cry more than firstborns, while firstborns show a tendency to smile more than only-born children. However, by 12 and 24 months, firstborn and only children do not show any reliable differences in their social behavior observed in a free-play lab setting. The cognitive performance of firstborn children is higher than onlies at 12 months, although by 24 months the two groups score similarly on the Bayley M DI. These results indicate that at least as infants, firstborn and only children may be different in their behavior, although these differences are not apparent later.

Firstborn children who are less fussy, more smiling, and more cognitively competent may have an impact on their parents' decision on whether or how soon to have another baby. It is possible that only-born children are as infants more "difficult" in temperament (cry more, smile less, are more irregular and less adaptive) or less cognitively reponsive and therefore prove a more demanding task for new parents, thus affecting the parents' decision to have a second child. While our data indicate onlies may be temperamentally more fussy as infants, by the time they are toddlers onlies are as sociable as firstborns and do not exhibit antisocial behaviors predicted by the negative only-child stereotype.

Differences in First and Only-Born Children
Related to Differences in Parents

Another possible source for differences in only and firstborn children is related to parental characteristics and behavior. The effect of parents on children has been a major theme in child development since its beginning (see Hartup, 1978; Lewis and Goldberg, 1969). Parents have been shown to influence their children's social (see Clarke-Stewart, 1973, 1978; Lamb, 1976; Lewis and Rosenblum, 1979) as well as cognitive development (see Lewis, 1976). Parental differences may take many forms, such as differences in demographic characteristics, personality, and beliefs, as well as parenting styles. Our data suggest that mothers of only and firstborn children may be different in their demographic characteristics and beliefs. Data from 3-month maternal interviews show that mothers of only borns report a smaller ideal family size, tend to feel less positive about becoming pregnant, and are less likely to have a normal pregnancy and delivery, as compared to mothers of firsts. In addition, mothers of onlies tended to be older at the birth of their children than mothers of firsts. Although the data do not enable us to make causal statements, they do suggest that mothers who desire smaller families may wait longer before they have a first child. It is also possible that having a child at a later age predisposes a person to having a more difficult childbearing experience and consequently adversely effects one's decision about whether or when to have a second child.

Parents of only and firstborn children also show a difference in parenting behavior. At 3 months mothers of onlies are more proximal in their behavior, rocking and kissing their infants more than do mothers of firstborns. At 12 months mothers of onlies are still more proximal in their behavior and also play more with their children, although mothers of firsts and onlies are similar in the other behaviors observed, such as smile, look, and vocalization. At 24 months mothers of onlies tend to show slightly more approval than do mothers of firsts; otherwise mothers are similar in their social behavior in the lab setting.

In general, focusing on differences, mothers of onlies appear more attentive to their young children in terms of proximal behavior at 3 and 12 months, as compared to mothers of firsts. Eidusons' (1976) suggestion that the most salient feature distinguishing the only child's socialization is that there is only one child to absorb parental interest and attention is supported and broadened by our findings. The fact that mothers of onlies were more attentive to their children than are mothers of firsts (who in fact were also mothers with only one child at the time of observation) suggests that only children may be the recipients of even more parental attention due to the special nature of their parents, even beyond the phenomena of the "overconcerned primaparous parent." At this point it should be noted that at 3 months only borns tended to cry more than firstborns and mothers of onlies showed more proximal caretaking activities. The nature of our data collection procedure makes it impossible to determine whether parents (due to some personality characteristics) are reinforcing child differences in crying or whether parents are responding to differences in their children's crying behavior, perhaps due to some temperament characteristic. It most probably is the case that both parent and child factors are contributing to the observed differences in only and firstborn groups.

Differences in First and Only-Born Children Related to the Birth of a Second Child

A third source of possible difference between only and firstborn children has to do with the birth and presence of a second child. In other words, firstborn children may be different from only-born children in that they experience the addition of another child into the family in which there was previously only one child. While only children may experience uninterrupted parental focus, firstborns must give up their parents' undivided attention upon the birth of a second child. For example, research by Dunn and Kendrick (1979, 1980) indicates that after the birth of a second child, firstborns show an increase in sleep disturbances and are more likely to make verbal demands of the mother following an interaction between the mother and the new baby.

Our findings, although based on a small sample, show that at 24 months those ten children who had acquired a sibling performed the lowest on the Bayley MDI, compared to firstborns who would acquire a sibling later, or only born children. This is in particular contrast to these ten children's 12-month data, in which they scored the highest on the Bayley. Thus, the results suggest that the birth and presence of a second child affects the firstborn child, and this may be a source of difference between first and only-born children. As Thompson (1974) suggests, firstborns' experience of "dethroning," an experience not shared by only borns, may be an important source of the difference between the behavior patterns of these groups. Our findings are also consistent with the work of Zajonc (1976), who predicts a lower intelligence score for those firstborn children who have a very young sibling when the average intelligence over all family members is lower by the infant sibling's presence.

SUMMARY

In summary, the data suggest that all three sources of variation — child characteristics, parent characteristics, and birth of a sibling — may affect observed differences in only and firstborn children. Differences in the temperament characteristics of firstborn and only children may be reflected in the early tendency of only infants to be more fussy, less sociable, and less cognitively alert than firstborn infants. Parents of only and firstborns may be different themselves and consequently treat and engender differences in their children. Mothers of onlies were older at the birth of the first child, expressed the desire for fewer children, and had a more difficult childbearing experience. In terms of parental behavior, mothers of onlies were more involved in their infants. Finally, the birth of a sibling was noted to change the cognitive performance of firstborn children in a negative way. This suggests that firstborn children are different from onlies as a result of experiencing the entrance of a new infant into the family.

Overall, the data suggest that although only borns may be more fussy as infants, this behavior does not persist into early childhood. The data gathered from free-play laboratory observation do not support the negative stereotype of the antisocial, self-centered only-born child. While mothers of only-born children seem more closely involved with their infants (as indicated by proximal behavior at 3 and 12 months), this maternal attention does not appear to engender a "spoiled child" phenomenon. Thus, the negative social consequences of being an only child predicted by the prevalent stereotype are not supported by the data we collected on mothers and children in the first two years of life.

REFERENCES

Bell, R. Q. Stimulus control of parent or caretaker behavior by offspring. *Developmental Psychology*, 1971, 4, 63-72.

Carey, W. B. A simplified method for measuring infant temperament. *Journal of Pediatrics*, 1970, 77, 188-194.

Chess, S., Thomas, A., and Cameron, M. Temperament: Its significance for early schooling. *New York University Education Quarterly.* Spring 1976, 24-29.

Clarke-Stewart, K. A. Interaction between mothers and their young children: Characteristics and consequences. *Monographs of the Society for Research in Child Development*, 1973, 38 (Serial No. 153).

Clarke-Stewart, K. A. And daddy makes three: The father's impact on mother and young child. *Child Development*, 1978, 49(2), 466-478.

Dunn, J., and Kendrick, C. Interaction between young siblings in the context of family relationships. In M. Lewis and L. Rosenblum (Eds.), *The child and its family: The genesis of behavior* (Vol. 2). New York: Plenum, 1979, 143-168.

Dunn, J., and Kendrick, C. The arrival of a sibling: Changes in patterns of interaction between mother and first born child. *Journal of Child Psychology and Psychiatry*, 1980, 21(2), 119-132.

Eiduson, B. T. *The dynamics of the one child family: Socialization implications.* Paper presented at the Symposium on the Only Child at the meetings of the American Psychological Association, Washington, D.C., September 1976.

Falbo, T. The only child: A review. *Journal of Individual Psychology*, 1977, 33(1), 47-61.

Falbo, T. Only children and interpersonal behavior: An experimental and survey study. *Journal of Applied Social Psychology*, forthcoming.

Feiring, C. *The influence of the child and secondary parent on maternal behavior toward a social systems' view of early infant-mother attachment.* Doctoral dissertation, University of Pittsburgh, 1975.

Gewirtz, J. L., and Gewirtz, H. B. Stimulus conditions, infant behaviors, and social learning in four Israeli childrearing environments: A preliminary report illustrating differences in environment and behavior between "only" and "youngest" child. In B. M. Foss (Ed.), *Determinants of infant behavior* (Vol. 3). New York: Wiley, 1965.

Gough, H. *The adjective checklist.* Palo Alto, CA: Consulting Psychologists Press, 1952.

Greenberg, M. S. Role playing: An alternative to deception? *Journal of Personality and Social Psychology*, 1967, 7(2), 152-157.

Harper, L. V. The scope of offspring effects: From caregiver to culture. *Psychological Bulletin*, 1975, 82, 784-801.

Hartup, W. W. Perspectives on child and family interaction: Past, present, and future. In R. M. Lerner and G. B. Spanier (Eds.), *Child influences on marital and family interaction: A life-span perspective.* New York: Academic Press, 1978, 23-42.

Hoyt, M. P., and Raven, B. H. Birth order and the 1971 Los Angeles earthquake. *Journal of Personality and Social Psychology*, 1973, 28(1), 123-128.

Lamb, M. E. (Ed.). *The role of the father in child development.* New York: Wiley, 1976.

Lewis, M. State an infant-environment interaction: An analysis of mother-infant interaction as a function of sex. *Merrill-Palmer Quarterly*, 1972, 18, 95-121.

Lewis, M. (Ed.). *The origins of intelligence: Infancy and early childhood.* New York: Plenum, 1976.

Lewis, M., and Goldberg, S. Perceptual-cognitive development in infancy: A generalized expectancy model as a function of the mother-infant interaction. *Merrill-Palmer Quarterly*, 1969, 15(1), 81-100.

Lewis, M., and Rosenblum, L. (Eds.). *The origins of fear: The origins of behavior* (Vol. 2). New York: Wiley, 1974.

Lewis, M., and Rosenblum, L. (Eds.). *The child and its family: The genesis of behavior* (Vol. 2). New York: Plenum, 1979.

Parke, R. D., and Sawin, D. B. Infant characteristics and behavior as elicitors of maternal and paternal responsiveness in the newborn period. Paper presented at the meetings of the Society for Research in Child Development, Denver, April 1975.

Pinner, B., and Thompson, V. D. *The taboo against the one-child family.* Unpublished manuscript, University of North Carolina at Chapel Hill, 1974.

Schachter, S. *The psychology of affiliation.* Stanford, CA: Stanford University Press, 1959.

Thompson, V. D. Family size: Implicit policies and assumed psychological outcomes. *Journal of Social Issues,* 1974, 30(4), 93-124.

Toman, W., and Toman, E. Sibling positions of a sample of distinguished persons. *Perceptual and Motor Skills,* 1970, 31(3), 825-826.

Zajonc, R. B. Family configuration and intelligence: Variations in scholastic aptitude scores parallel trends in family size and the spacing of children. *Science,* 1976, 192, 227-236.

9

Work and Fertility

James A. Sweet

The last fifteen years have been a very active period for scholars interested in the interconnections between the employment of women and fertility. Developments in theory, data availability, and statistical method have interacted to lead us toward a more thorough understanding of reproductive and labor force processes and the interconnections between them. At the same time, there have been significant changes in American society. The education level is greater for each successive cohort. The family and other major social institutions are undergoing transformation. The baby-boom cohorts have reached adulthood and, because of their large size, face a scarcity of employment opportunity. Some argue that our basic values have changed, using terms such as the "me generation" to describe these major shifts in social values. There have been important developments in birth-control technology and practice, and we are close to the point where our reproduction is under control. The women's

SOME OF the ideas in this chapter were first presented in a paper, "The Sociological Analysis of Low Fertility," coauthored with Larry Bumpass and presented at the 1980 meetings of the American Sociological Association. My thinking on the subjects of employment and fertility and the relationships between them has benefited greatly from my association and collaboration in teaching and research with Larry Bumpass. Linda Jacobsen provided valuable comments on the manuscript. The preparation of the chapter was supported by Grant HD-11366 from the Center for Population Research of the National Institute of Child Health and Human Development.

movement has developed and has led us to be more accepting, if not encouraging, of nonfamilial roles for women, and to institute important legal changes in the status of women. In addition, a new emphasis on environmental quality has led many to question whether the high levels of reproduction characteristic of the postwar baby-boom period are desirable or even socially tolerable. These important social changes have affected both employment patterns and reproductive patterns of American women, as well as the relationship between work and reproduction.

In this chapter I will review some of the major issues with respect to work and fertility that have received the attention of social scientists in recent years. I will describe several alternative theoretical and conceptual approaches to these issues, and will make some suggestions concerning fruitful directions of future research.

PERSPECTIVES ON THE RELATIONSHIP BETWEEN EMPLOYMENT AND FERTILITY

There are several different perspectives from which employment patterns and reproductive patterns of women have been investigated. To some extent these perspectives correspond to disciplinary boundaries, but to a large extent they are independent of academic discipline.

(1) normative perspective, deriving from sociology

(2) time-allocation perspective, deriving from economics

(3) work and career commitment or sex role socialization perspective, deriving from social psychology

(4) life-cycle or experiential perspective, deriving from social demography

There are few pure examples of empirical or theoretical work that fit entirely within one or another of these categories. Most recent work is a hybrid drawing on two or more of these perspectives. Each of them offers considerable insight into reproductive and employment behavior, recent changes in these behaviors, and the causal connections between them.

Normative Perspective

This perspective emphasizes the normative pressures on women in American society to place the highest priority on reproduction and motherhood. Social norms are shared beliefs concerning what is appropriate behavior. Norms are supported by a set of sanctions that reward conformity and punish deviation. Society tends to socialize individual members so that they behave in conformity with the norms, more or less automatically. The normative perspective begins with the premise that to be a woman in American society is to be a wife and a mother. These roles are predominant. Other roles are appropriate only to the extent that they do not interfere, in any appreciable way, with the spousal and maternal roles.

The key concept in much of sociological theory of fertility is the reproductive norm and the normative pressures to reproduce. It is important to appreciate that this theory was developed during the baby-boom period, when a high, seemingly dysfunctional, level of fertility was what needed to be understood. According to this theory, family size norms guide the behavior of individual members of society to ensure that reproductive levels are in equilibrium with, or appropriate to, the social structure, the technology, and the environment. The number of offspring that an individual couple chooses to have is influenced both by their assessment of the number of children appropriate to the objective social and economic conditions in which they find themselves and by the social norm concerning how many children are regarded as appropriate.

Ryder (1979: 361) has summarized his understanding of the content of American fertility norms:

> Social norms in the United States, at least until recently, have pressed people into a preference for marriage over nonmarriage, parenthood over nonparenthood, and at least two children rather than only one — with the proviso that one should be in a position to fulfill one's parental obligations. Beyond the second child, the progression is primarily a matter of individual preference, although friends, neighbors, and relatives may look askance if the number goes beyond four.

Norms are not simply another "cost" or "factor" to be taken into account when making reproductive decisions. They are not simply another variable to take into account in multivariate analyses of fertility differences among couples. Instead, they are "built into" the social structure of a society and into the personalities of its members. Because they are institutionalized and socialized into personality, they are not likely to change rapidly or be much influenced by short-term changes in economic and social conditons. This is not to say that they are eternally fixed, but rather that change will occur slowly and only as a concomitant of rather fundamental social change.

There are many excellent sociological discussions of the societal pressures on women and couples to marry and reproduce. Nancy Russo (1976) has discussed the "Motherhood Mandate." Ellen Peck and others involved in the "nonparent movement" have discussed the pressures on young people to become parents, and have given advice on how to resist them (see Peck and Sanderowitz, 1974). Judith Blake (1972) uses the term "coercive pronatalism" to describe the ubiquitous social pressures to marry and reproduce. Similar ideas are discussed by Betty Friedan (1965) in *The Feminine Mystique* and Jessie Bernard (1975) in *The Future of Motherhood*.

Strangely, there are few explicit discussions of whether and how fertility norms may be changing. The only statement that we could find is a very cautious one of Ryder. He suggests (1979: 361) that the baby boom can be explained without reference to changing values: "The steady rise in real income, together with increasing governmental intervention which effectively transferred resources away from nonparents and toward parents, made feasible the almost universal adherence to a long-standing norm of proper behavior." However, with reference to the past decade-and-a-half, Ryder (1979: 361) admits that it is difficult to explain the rapidly rising proportion with fewer than two children: "Perhaps we must consider the possibility that the norms themselves may be changing — that motherhood is becoming less a matter of obligation and more a matter of preference."

What does this normative perspective imply about employment and the relationship between employment and fertility? Not only are there pressures on women to marry and bear children; there are also social pressures on women to be good mothers, in the sense of caring for and socializing their children. If possible, women should be full-time mothers, at least until their youngest child is in school, and preferably until the child has reached high school age or beyond.

There have been several studies of public opinion on these matters. In 1965, Morgan et al. (1966) asked a sample of household heads a question: "Suppose a family has children, but they are all in school. Would you say it is a good thing for the wife to take a job, a bad thing, or what?" Nearly half of the predominantly male sample responded unfavorably to the question, and about one-third gave favorable responses.

Retert and Bumpass (1974) analyzed a series of questions asked in 1970 of white mothers with children under the age of four. Seventeen percent approved of the mother of an infant working. Three-quarters felt that preschoolers are harmed by the mother working, and 89 percent reported that their husbands preferred that they not work.

Work is inappropriate to the extent that it interferes with being a "good" wife and mother. Husbands expect their wives to take care of their families. Society expects that adult women marry, bear children, care for husbands and children, and maintain the household. Work outside the home is acceptable only if it does not interfere with these familial functions, or when it is absolutely necessary in order for the family to maintain a minimal standard of living.

Some corollaries of this perspective are the following:

(1) Women's employment rates will vary over the life cycle. Work will be "fit in" when possible, or necessary, during periods when childcare is less intense.

(2) Women workers are typically sporadic workers. They may work for periods of time when their families are in particularly great economic need and/or when childcare responsibilities are small, but they will be unlikely to be persistent workers.

(3) Women will choose occupations in which continuity of employment is relatively unimportant (see Polachek, 1979).

(4) Women will avoid jobs that require a commitment and a willingness to work long or odd hours, those jobs involving travel, and those requiring residential mobility.

(5) Women will tend to choose jobs that use the same skills and temperament appropriate to mothering — patience, nurturance, and so on (see Oppenheimer, 1970).

Allocation of Time

A second perspective is that of many economists, which emphasizes the allocation of time. Time is a scarce resource. Every individual has only twenty-four hours a day, seven days a week, fifty-two weeks a year. This time must be allocated among a whole array of activities, including maintaining one's self (sleeping, eating, bathing), work, recreation, socialization and care of the young, and so forth. Time is scarce and has economic value.

The basic idea of this economic perspective on fertility is that children may be viewed, in effect, as consumer durables, such as automobiles or sailboats, from which parents derive pleasure or utility. Because of this value, parents are willing to pay the costs associated with childrearing: direct financial costs associated with feeding, clothing, and maintaining children for two decades or so; the opportunity costs of the parents' time; and the other "psychic" costs of coexisting in a household with children experiencing the "terrible twos" or the strains of adolescence. (For nontechnical discussions of the economic perspective on family decisions see Sawhill, 1977; Smith, 1979; and Turchi, 1975.) As costs increase, parents demand fewer children; as incomes rise, parents will demand more children. Presumably, as the pleasure or utility derived from children changes, the number of children "demanded" will also change, although investigation of this aspect of the process has not been a major concern of economists.

In evaluating the "costs" of children, one of the major components is the opportunity costs of earnings foregone by the mother. According to the estimates of Espenshade (1977),

> the direct cost of raising a child from birth to age 18 ranged from $35,000 to $54,000 (in 1977 dollars). When the average cost of four years of college is added to this the cost rises to $44,000-$64,000. In addition the opportunity cost of wages foregone by the mother adds an average of $35,000 to this total for a first child. The opportunity cost of subsequent children is considerably smaller. The opportunity cost component is higher, the higher the education of the mother, since wage rates increase with education.

Of course, many mothers interrupt employment for only a brief period, if at all, at the time of childbirth and continue to work outside the home full-time and continuously through childrearing years (see Bumpass and Sweet, 1980). How can such a woman be said to have "foregone" earnings? Clearly, she has not. However, the economic model says that she has foregone "leisure," or that time was spent rearing those children that could have been spent in other leisure (nonwork) pursuits. It is reasonable to evaluate the time spent in leisure in terms of the market value of the woman's time — her hourly wage rate. This implies that the greater the potential earnings of a woman, the more expensive it is for her to have a child (see Butz and Ward, 1977, 1979a, 1979b).

Sex Role or Work Commitment Perspective

Related to the "normative perspective" is what I will call a "sex role" or "work-commitment" perspective. The distinction between them rests primarily on the level of analysis. The normative perspective is primarily macrosociological. The sex role or work-commitment perspective is more psychological, focusing on individual variation in orientations. Kupinsky (1977: 223) summarizes this perspective:

> The more modern, instrumental and individualistic her sex-role orientation, the more likely a married women is to perceive the economic and psychological benefits of working as greater than the economic and psychological benefits of bearing and rearing children, and thus to be more strongly committed to her worker role and to restrict her family size. Conversely, the more traditional, family-centered her sex-role orientation, the more likely she is to perceive the economic and psychological benefits of childbearing and rearing as greater than the benefits of working, the less likely she is to be committed to the worker role if she were to enter the labor force and the greater the liklihood that she would have more children than the modern-oriented, work-committed woman.

Thus, modernity or traditionalism of sex role orientations is causally related to both work and fertility and produces the association between the two behaviors. Examples of work from this perspective include that of Scanzoni (1975), who contrasts sex role modernity or an "instrumental" or individualistic orientation with a sex role-traditional or more expressive orientation, and of Mason (1974), who distinguishes "role-modern" women, who emphasize achievement, from "role-traditional" women, who emphasize familism.

There is a related perspective which emphasizes work commitment or career orientation. Women with a greater work commitment or career orientation are more likely to be working and to have restricted fertility than those with less. Much of the empirical work taking this approach uses a rather questionable circular measure of work commitment, the amount of prior work experience (see Kupinsky, 1971, and Mason, 1974, for a critique.) It seems that if work commitment or career orientation are invoked as operative in the work-fertility relationship, they need to be measured prior to, and independently of, the work experience (and reproductive behavior) they seek to explain.

It is evident that (if properly measured) individual women do vary in their degrees of work commitment or career orientation. This commitment is somehow a product of early socialization. Women with high degrees of work orientation will place higher priority on employment, will presumably have fewer children, and will be more likely to work given the ages and numbers of children and other objective factors. An important focus of research would seek to identify the aspects of early socialization that affect the relative emphasis on work and reproduction. For example, did the woman's mother work? How many children were in her family of orientation? What educational experiences did she have that contributed to an achievement orientation? Other research seeks to identify the sources of variation in sex role orientations (what is appropriate for men and women to do) and the effects of these prior sex role orientations on women's work and reproductive behavior. These concerns are similar to some of those that motivated the original 1941 Indianapolis fertility study (Kiser and Whelpton, 1958) and the Princeton Study of family growth in metropolitan America (Westoff et al., 1961, 1963).

Life-Cycle/Experiential Perspective

The final perspective on work-fertility relationships is what I would call a life-cycle/experiential model. This perspective on work and fertility is part of a general trend in sociology, and in social demography in particular, toward adopting a more dynamic perspective on life-cycle processes. It recognizes that the various spheres of life are interconnected with one another. Reproductive behavior, for example, must be viewed within the context of the career development (or lack thereof) of husbands, the work experience of women, the experience of marriage and childrearing, and the changing economic resources and obligations that confront the family unit. Neither reproductive plans nor work and career plans are fixed over time. Both vary in reponse to the changing objective conditions and experiences of both husband and wife.

Women's fertility goals and their work orientation are products of both early socialization and their experiences as they proceed through the family life cycle. Experience with work may change work or fertility orientations. So, too, may experience with childrearing. Changes in the economic position of a couple or in their standard of living — their desired lifestyle — may also modify reproductive and employment orientations. Particularly important may be early adult experience — young women living on their own neither in family of orientation nor in a married status, for instance. Early work experience — both its quantity and its quality — may affect these orientations.

I will discuss some issues of particular relevance to this last perspective in later sections. I will illustrate this perspective with several examples.

Veevers (1973) has studied the experience of voluntarily childless couples. The most striking common theme in the experience of her sample of childless couples was that they started out planning to have children but for various reasons postponed their first birth. Eventually their lives developed in ways that led to a decision to remain childless.

Waite (1980b) has shown that the relationship between wife's employment and education, potential wage rate, and family economic conditions varies depending on "life-cycle stage." For example, the employment rate of women who have had all the children that they intend to have is more responsive to family economic circumstances than that of young women who have not yet had children or those mothers who plan to have additional births (see also Sweet, 1973: Ch. 5).

Oppenheimer (1974, 1979) has emphasized what she terms "life-cycle squeezes," which put economic pressure on wives to work. The first occurs early in marriage, as the young couple establishes a household. At this time there is need for considerable capital investment in household equipment at a time when young husbands are at the beginning of their careers and tend to have low earnings. The second "squeeze" occurs when adolescent and college-age children are present in the home. The costs of maintaining children at these ages are very high, and husbands tend to have earnings levels that have already peaked, or at least are not increasing very rapidly.

Oppenheimer also emphasizes that there are variations by husband's occupation in the timing and severity of these squeezes.

CAUSAL RELATIONSHIP BETWEEN FERTILITY AND LABOR FORCE PARTICIPATION

There has been a whole series of studies attempting to model statistically the causal relationship between employment and fertility. These studies have used a wide variety of measures of work and fertility and various methodologies. A discussion of this literature is provided by Waite (1980a, 1980b). Some examples of this work include that of Willis (1973), Waite and Stolzenberg (1976), Stolzenberg and Waite (1977), Smith-Lovin and Tickamyer (1978), Hout (1978), and Cramer (1980).

The causal relationship between employment and fertility is difficult to assess. Numerous studies demonstrate that the more children a woman has borne or intends to bear, the lower her employment probability. However, this association does not demonstrate the causal ordering:

(1) Women who wish to work may restrict their fertility in order to pursue more easily their career objectives.

(2) Women who wish to bear children may restrict their employment in order to devote more time to childrearing activities.

(3) Women who are subfecund, or who restrict their fertility for other reasons, may work with greater frequency simply because there are fewer children to make demands on their time or otherwise constrain their decisions.

(4) Work and fertility behaviors may be related to each other only because they are causally associated with other characteristics, such as education or certain psychological characteristics.

(5) Work and fertility in the economist's schema are likely to be associated in a complex reciprocal relationship. For an individual, certain tastes and background characteristics affect a woman's education, marriage age, and early work experience. The woman's wage rate and work experience are determined by these factors. Her fertility, in turn, is affected by all these factors, including the opportunity cost of childbearing in terms of earnings foregone during her absence from the labor force. The entire process occurs, in the case of married women, within a family context in which the

wage rate, earnings, and "tastes" of a husband (and perhaps other household members) are also relevant.

Although numerous studies have attempted to develop a causal model of this complex reality, none has to date done a totally convincing job. The problem is only partially one of data or statistical limitations. Rather, the complexity of the process is beyond our capacity to conceptualize and model. Both work experience and fertility experience are the outcome of cumulative processes that begin at birth (within the family of orientation, and social and economic background) and continue through the life cycle. Each transition in the process is conditioned by prior experience in various spheres of life and by the social and economic context within which the woman is currently living.

It has long been a dictum that we require longitudinal data in order to tease out the causal associations among work experience, sex role attitudes, and fertility. In addition to these longitudinal studies, there have been efforts to collect retrospective fertility and employment histories and to develop procedures for their analysis. New statistical modeling techniques have been applied to this problem.

Recently a great deal of effort has gone into searching for *the* relationship between employment and fertility. There seems to be an abiding faith that if we were only able to ask the right survey questions (preferably in a longitudinal study), with the right, nonrecursive statistical method, we would finally be able to estimate the "right" model, get the "true" reciprocal coefficients, and know once and for all the relative size of the reciprocal effects.

I am not suggesting that this effort has been wasted, that newly applied statistical modeling procedures are not useful, or that longitudinal designs are not helpful in teasing out these complex relationships. Rather, what I would emphasize is that there are numerous dimensions to the work-fertility relationship, and it will be necessary to continue to chip away at understanding these various processes. I doubt that there is either a statistical "fix" or an ideal set of survey questions that will resolve the question once and for all. Even if there were an "answer" to the question of the relative size of these reciprocal effects, there would remain a lot of unanswered questions of great import about the underlying processes. Continuing to seek *the* relationship between work and fertility is not likely to be fruitful.

Attention should be directed at understanding the numerous processes that relate employment and reproductive behavior.

WORK AND FERTILITY IN THE LIFE CYCLE: NEEDED RESEARCH

In the balance of this chaper, I will discuss three aspects of the relationship between work and fertility that seem to me to deserve further attention of sociologists, economists, and social demographers. These are:

(1) the processes by which the age at entry into marriage and parenthood affects reproductive and work decisions;

(2) the processes by which the "quality" of a woman's employment, as distinct from the mere fact of whether she is employed or not, affects subsequent reproductive and employment decisions; and

(3) the processes by which the economic conditions faced by young adults, prior to and early in their marriages, affect employment, marriage, and reproductive decisions.

Age at Entry into Marriage and Motherhood

One of the persisting fertility differentials is the inverse relationship between age at marriage and fertility. Particularly women who marry in their teens have considerably higher fertility than those who marry in their twenties. Further, persons who marry at young ages tend to have higher rates of marital disruption.

In the past decade or so, much attention has been given to the long-term effects of early motherhood on the life chances of women. It is now well established that women who marry at young ages and/or bear their first children at young ages have more children during their lifetimes and have their subsequent births at more rapid intervals. Their life chances also appear to be adversely affected in a variety of ways (see Baldwin, 1976).

It has often been observed that "later means fewer," and we regard the combination of rising marriage ages and increased delay of birth within marriage as of profound significance. Yet there has been rather little attention of questions to the processes by which delays affect subsequent reproductive behavior. There are several more or less distinct processes operating, several of which are related to employment.

Women who spend an increasing period of time "on their own" (outside of the parental household and not in a marital relationship) may form a rather different "self-image" and set of opinions about the roles appropriate for women in general and for themselves in particular. Mason (1974) refers to the significance of a "role hiatus" as an influence on sex role attitudes and "tastes" for work:

> Because most women in this society operate within a role-traditional milieu, the extent to which their personal sex-role conceptions or relative tastes for work deviate from the traditional model will depend on having non-traditional experiences prior to the formation of a family. Women who live for some period as neither "daughters," "wives," nor "mothers" should, in other words, be more likely to establish outlooks which conflict with the traditional image of the "selfless" helpmate woman than will those going from one relatively dependent status to another without break. Women experiencing role hiatuses are also likely to have stronger tastes for work, especially if their "role hiatus" experiences expose them to or emphasize some form of occupationally relevant, individualistic activity.

Under the baby-boom fertility pattern, marriage could almost be equated with parenthood, since reproduction began immediately after marriage for most couples. It seems likely that marital relationships develop differently when they do not begin almost immediately with pregnancy and parenthood. It appears rather important to trace the ways in which a delay of first birth may modify the relationship between partners in ways that in turn affect subsequent fertility. Again, issues of self-image and appropriate adult roles and employment patterns of both husbands and wives may be involved.

Similarly, couples are likely to become involved in a different set of leisure activities in the absence of children from what they would have as parents. These constitute new lifestyle opportunity costs that might not have been as salient when marriage was followed immediately by pregnancy and parenthood.

As marriages are delayed, and births within marriage further delayed, it seems likely that the timing of the first birth, and in fact whether to have a birth at all, may become more of a matter to be considered in something approximating cost-benefit terms than simply a concomitant of marriage. The same may be true of subsequent births.

Most of the discussions of the implications of delay of marriage and motherhood emphasize that women have more of an opportunity to gain work experience at young ages. The resulting greater "commitment" to market work and greater earning potential increase the opportunity cost of subsequent childbearing (see Polachek, 1975: Sandell and Shapiro, 1978).

A related but somewhat distinct idea is that the couple may establish a living standard based on two incomes, which requires the wife either to restrict fertility or to commit herself to the combination of childrearing, housework, and market work. While childrearing and housekeeping tasks may be shared by the husband, the burden still falls disproportionately on the wife in the current setting.

We need to explore further how increased work experience among young women affects subsequent reproductive decisions, how early fertility experience affects subsequent employment patterns, and how couples adjust the organization of housework, childrearing, and market work. We need to know more about the process of adapting lifestyles to the arrival of the first and subsequent births and to the exit and entry of wives in the labor force. With a majority of wives, and now even a majority of mothers, working in paid employment it should be clear that one major "cost" of children must be the cost of leisure foregone. We have little understanding of how parents and prospective parents perceive this cost of childbearing or what adjustments are made in "leisure" activities as the first, and subsequent, children are added to a family. It seems clear that more attention ought to be paid to time use and particularly leisure time use as it relates to reproductive decisions.

Quality of Women's Employment

One important distinction that has received little attention in the work-fertility literature is that between the quantity and quality of women's employment experience. Rates of female employment have increased dramatically in the United States over the past forty years or more. By the end of the 1970s over half of all adult women were in the labor force. Some of the rise in employment rates has been due to rising educational levels and to changes in the distribution of family status (marital status, presence and ages of children). Most of it, however, is independent of changing population composition (Sweet, 1979a).

It is no longer reasonable to categorize American wives into workers and nonworkers. Such a division is appropriate to classify a woman's current employment status, but in a longer time perspective virtually all wives work at some time during the life cycle. However, it is equally erroneous to regard working women as typically pursuing "careers" in the usual sense of the word — that is, in a position within an ordered sequence of positions through which one can normally expect to progress during one's worklife. Most women are in occupations in which there is little prospect for upward mobility. To the extent that they are in occupations in which there are mobility opportunities, women tend to face discrimination in promotion or are unable to respond to opportunities for promotion because of constraints, such as being unable or unwilling to relocate in another community (because husbands' jobs are regarded as more important than wives' jobs) or being unwilling to accept jobs involving travel or irregular hours (because of family demands). A woman of a given age typically has less seniority than a male of the same age because of interruptions in worklife due to childbearing or residential mobility associated with the husband's career. Further, the labor market processes that result in occupation segregation also place women disproportionately in occupations with relatively few supervisory positions; for example, there are many school teachers and very few principals. Wolf and Fligstein (1979a, 1979b) have documented a sex differential in "authority" that is independent of education or occupational status. Hence, mobility opportunities are very restricted.

There has been little, if any, decrease in occupational segregation by sex. Women are concentrated primarily in "women's jobs" and men in "men's jobs." This was true a half-century ago, and it is true today. Not only has there been little change in occupational segregation in recent years (Williams, 1979); there has also been no improvement in the occupational standing of young women. Young women were *less* likely to be in an occupation commensurate with their education in 1976 than in 1970, and were less likely in 1970 than in 1960 (Sweet, 1979b).

The earnings of women are about two-thirds those of men after appropriate controls (Fuchs, 1971), and there is no evidence of improvement in this fraction. The sex differential in earnings is largely attributed to occupational segregation by sex. Some, but probably not a majority, of the male-female earnings difference is due to the fact that women accrue less work experience by any given age than do men (Mincer and Polachek, 1974; Sandell and Shapiro, 1978). The earnings of men increase with age and experience, while those of women are more nearly invariant with age (see Kohen, 1975; Sexton, 1977).

What would happen to reproductive levels if women's postion in the labor market were to improve to the point that opportunities for women were more nearly equal to those for men? Is it likely that considerably larger numbers of women would choose to remain child-less, or to have only one child? Perhaps, given the lack of progress in recent decades, it is frivolous to ask such a question. On the other hand, there are reasons that the next few decades may see significant improvements. Recently, there has been increasing public concern for the equality of opportunity of women in the United States. Both legislation and judicial decisions have restricted the degree to which employers may discriminate on the basis of sex. In addition, the lack of progress toward equality in the economy in recent decades must be seen in the context of changes in the supply of young workers in general and of female workers in particular. The size of the population, its age structure, educational change, and the rising rate of labor force participation have all resulted in very rapidly growing numbers of workers competing for available jobs (see Smith and Welch, 1978).

Easterlin (1978) and other economists emphasize the effect of cohort size on the economic position of young males. This pronatalist effect of decreasing cohort size must be tempered with a recognition that a decreasing supply of new workers competing for positions and other social processes for equality of economic opportunity for women could result in marked reduction in occupational segregation by sex and a major improvement in the position of women in the labor market. This could have a significant antinatalist effect. Past experience with increases in the fraction of women working, with no improvement in the quality of work, does not give us much of a basis for predicting the effect on fertility of such a change.

Recent Trends in the Economic Conditions of the Early Years of Marriage

In considering the economics of reproductive decisions, it is important to focus attention on the early years of marriage. This is especially the case when considering fertility change during the 1970s. I have examined the recent changes in the economic circumstances of young couples (Sweet, 1979c, 1980). The data show quite clearly that the earnings of young men rose continuously during the 1950s and 1960s. During periods of recesssions the rate of increase slowed, but the trend was clearly upward. During the 1970s, however, the trend was different. There were wide fluctuations in the real earnings of young husbands, and there was no continued upward trend. Even when we consider the total income of couples, there was very little improvement. More wives had earnings, and those with earnings had higher earnings, but this simply kept couple income from declining. This cessation of growth in the income of young couples was true at all educational levels. In fact, only the upgrading in the educational composition kept aggregate couple incomes from deteriorating.

Greater attention should be paid to the details of the economic conditions young couples face during the early years of marraige. There is evidence that young couples with relatively prosperous husbands accelerate reproduction (Rindfuss and Sweet, 1977; Rindfuss and MacDonald, 1980; MacDonald and Rindfuss, 1980). In addition to questions concerning the size, stability, and composition of couple income (husband's versus wife's earnings), more attention to the role of asset accumulation, consumer debt, mortgage debt, and expenditure patterns (reflecting life style) would be useful.

The relative indifference to these questions is reflected in the fact that few data sources on income, expenditures, or assets include questions on marriage duration or reproductive patterns, while data sets including marriage duration seem systematically to avoid gathering data on these economic conditions.

The emphasis on the economics of the early years of marriage is supported by Frejka's (1980) account of the success of recent pronatalist policy in Czechoslovakia, which involves loans to newlyweds and maternity grants and extended maternity leaves in an attempt to focus resources more directly on young couples as they are at the point of making reproductive decisions.

In addition, future fertility studies should pay more serious attention to housing needs and aspirations in their own right, as a motivation for restricting fertility and a pressure for women to work, as well as a component of the financial circumstances of early marriage.

Discussions of population policy, and of policies affecting population, particularly in Europe, inevitably get around to discussions of the deficiencies in the housing stock. Often the generalization is made, or at least implied, that a severe housing shortage has a marked antinatalist effect.

There has been both scholarly and journalistic speculation that the housing stock of the future will include a much larger share of multi-unit structures and that single-family units will be smaller and compactly spaced. Some analysts see high energy costs leading to a return of the population to urban centers or at least the cessation of growth of more remote peripheral areas. The relationship between housing supply (including various amenities associated with housing) and reproductive behavior needs to be further explored. One crucial dimension of housing is homeownership. Masnick et al. (1978) have observed:

> Homeownership has always been an important part of the American way of life. Family-building goals are often intertwined with aspirations to achieve the privacy, autonomy, economic stability and sense of pride that homeownership promises.

Discussions of high, baby-boom fertility have emphasized the significance of the postwar ease of acquiring a home of one's own in encouraging earlier marriage and accelerated reproduction. Continued increases in prices of single-family housing, high interest rates, high energy prices, and tightening of credit may make it more difficult for young couples to get into their own homes and provide pressures on wives to work more continuously. This may add to the delay in childbearing and lead to the reassessment of reproductive aims.

CONCLUSION

In this chapter, I have described recent trends in fertility and in the employment of women in the United States. I have reviewed several perspectives from which social scientists view fertility behavior and the employment behavior of women and the interconnections between them. I made several major points.

First, the relationship between work and fertility is many-faceted. Work and fertility decisions are affected by a variety of background and socialization factors, but they are also influenced by the experiences that women and their spouses have, particularly during the young adult years. Social scientists working from a variety of perspectives have made considerable headway in understanding these processes.

Second, I have questioned the value of attempting to model the relationship between work and fertility "as a whole." Instead, I expressed a preference for a research strategy that disaggregates the process into parts and examines the dynamics of the component parts. Several examples of fruitful research directions were discussed.

Third, one point that I did not make as explicitly as I might have is that the dynamics of employment and fertility decisions are probably not the same today as they were a decade or two ago. They are not likely to be the same at the turn of the next century as they are today. For example, Cherlin (1980) has documented an abrupt increase in the fraction of young women who expect to be working when they reach age 40. The sense of what is "appropriate" behavior for men and women has changed. For an assortment of reasons, childbearing has probably become much more a subject of cost-benefit calculation than was the case in the past. This suggests that we should be concerned not only with understanding the processes that relate work and fertility, but also with how these processes differ among successive cohorts.

REFERENCES

Baldwin, W. H. Adolescent pregnancy and childbearing — Growing concerns for Americans. (Population Reference Bureau) *Population Bulletin*, 1976, 31(2), 1-34.

Bernard, J. *The future of motherhood*. New York: Dial, 1975.

Blake, J. Coercive pronatalism and American population policy. In R. Parke, Jr., and C. Westoff (Eds.), *Aspects of population growth policy*. U.S. Commission on Population Growth and the American Future Reports, Vol. 6. Washington, DC: Government Printing Office, 1972, 81-109.

Bumpass, L. L. and Sweet, J. A. *Patterns of employment before and after childbirth* (Vital and Health Statistics Series 23, No. 4. DHEW Publication [PHS] 80-1980). Hyattsville, MD: National Center for Health Statistics, 1980.

Butz, W. P., and Ward, M. P. The emergence of countercyclical U.S. fertility (Rand Paper R-1605-NIH). Santa Monica, CA: Rand Corporation, 1977.

Butz, W. P., and Ward, M. P. Will U.S. fertility remain low? A new economic interpretation. *Population and Development Review*, December 1979, 663-688. (a)

Butz, W. P., and Ward, M. P. Baby boom and baby bust: A new view. *American Demographics*, September 1979, 11-17. (b)

Cherlin, A. Postponing marriage: The influence of young women's work expectations. *Journal of Marriage and the Family*, 1980, 42(2), 355.

Cramer, J. C. Fertility and female employment: Problems of causal direction. *American Sociological Review*, April 1980, 167-190.

Easterlin, R. What will 1984 be like? Socioeconomic implications of recent twists in age structure. *Demography*, 1978, 15(4), 397-432.

Espenshade, T. The value and the cost of children. *Population Bulletin*, 1977, 32(1), 3-47. (Population Reference Bureau).

Friedan, B. *The feminine mystique*. New York: Dell, 1965.

Frejka, T. Fertility trends and policies: Czechoslovakia in the 1970s. Center for Policy Studies Working Paper 54 (February). New York: Population Council, 1980.

Fuchs, V. R. Differences in hourly earnings between men and women. *Monthly Labor Review*, 1971, 94(5), 9-15.

Hout, M. The determinants of marital fertility in the United States, 1968-70: Inferences from a dynamic model. *Demography*, 1978, 15, 139-60.

Kiser, C. V., and Whelpton, P. K. Social and psychological factors affecting fertility. *Milbank Memorial Fund Quarterly*, 1958, 36(3), 282-329.

Kohen, A. I., Breinich, S. C., and Shields, P. Women and the economy: A bibliography and a review of the literature on sex differentiation in the labor market. Columbus: Center for Human Resource Research, Ohio State University, 1975.

Kupinsky, S. Non-familial activity and socio-economic differentials in fertility. *Demography*, 1971, 8, 353-67.

Kupinsky, S. The fertility of working women in the United States: Historical trends and theoretical perspectives. In S. Kupinsky (Ed.), *The fertility of working women*. New York: Praeger, 1977.

MacDonald, M. M., and Rindfuss, R. R. Earnings, relative income, and family formation, 1977. Part I: Marriage (IRP Discussion Paper 615:80). Madison: Institute for Research on Poverty, University of Wisconsin, 1980.

Masnick, G., Wiget, B., Pitkin, J., and Myers, D. A life course perspective on the downturn in U.S. fertility (Center for Population Studies Working Paper 106). Cambridge, MA: Harvard University, 1978.

Mason, K. O. Women's labor force participation and fertility. Final Report 21U-662, prepared for the National Institutes of Health under contract NIH 71-2212, 1974.

Mincer, J., and Polachek, S. Family investments in human capital: Earnings of women. *Journal of Political Economy*, 1974, 82(2), S76-S108.

Morgan, J., Sirageldin, I., and Baerwaldt, N. *Productive Americans: A study of how individuals contribute to economic growth*. Ann Arbor: Institute for Social Research, University of Michigan, 1966.

Oppenheimer, V. K. *The female labor force in the United States*. Berkeley: Institute of International Studies, University of California, 1970.

Oppenheimer, V. K. The life-cycle squeeze: The interaction of men's occupational and family life cycles. *Demography*, 1974, 11(2), 227-245.

Oppenheimer, V. K. Structural sources of economic pressure for wives to work: an analytical framework. *Journal of Family History*, Summer 1979, 177.

Peck, E., and Sanderowitz, J. *Pronatalism: The myth of mom and apple pie*. New York: Thomas Y. Crowell, 1974.

Polachek, S. W. Discontinuous labor force participation and its effect on women's market earnings. In C. B. Lloyd (Ed.), *Sex, discrimination, and the division of labor*. New York: Columbia University Press, 1975, 90-122.

Polachek, S. W. Occupational segregation among women: Theory, evidence, and a prognosis. In C. B. Lloyd, E. S. Andrews, and C. L. Gilroy (Eds.), *Women in the labor market*. New York: Columbia University Press, 1979, 137-157.

Retert, S., and Bumpass, L. Employment and approval of employment among mothers of young children (CDE Working Paper 74-4). Madison: Center for Demography and Ecology, University of Wisconsin, 1974.

Rindfuss, R. R., and MacDonald, M. M. Earnings, relative income, and family formation, Part II: Fertility (IRP Discussion Paper 616-80). Madison: Institute for Research on Poverty, University of Wisconsin, 1980.

Rindfuss, R. R., and Sweet, J. A. *Postwar fertility trends and differentials in the United States.* New York: Academic Press, 1977.

Russo, N. The motherhood mandate. *Journal of Social Issues,* 1976, 32(3) 143-153.

Ryder, N. B. The future of American fertility. *Social Problems,* 1979, 26(3), 359-370.

Sandell, S. H., and Shapiro, D. The theory of human capital and the earnings of women: A re-examination of the evidence. *Journal of Human Resources,* 1978, 13(1), 103-117.

Sawhill, I. Economic perspectives on the family. *Daedalus,* 1977, 106(2), 115-125.

Scanzoni, J. H. *Sex roles, life styles, and childbearing: Changing patterns in marriage and the family.* New York: Free Press, 1975.

Sexton, P. C. *Women and work* (RD Monograph 46). Washington, DC: U.S. Department of Labor, Employment and Training Administration, 1977.

Smith, J. P., and Welch, F. The overeducated American? A review article (Rand Paper P-6253). Santa Monica, CA: Rand Corporation, 1978.

Smith, R. E. (Ed.), *The subtle revolution: Women at work.* Washington, DC: The Urban Institute, 1979.

Smith-Lovin, L., and Tickamyer, A. R. Labor force participation, fertility behavior, and sex attitudes. *American Sociological Review,* 1978, 43, 541-556.

Stolzenberg, R. M., and Waite, L. J. Age, fertility expectations, and plans for employment. *American Sociological Review,* 1977, 42, 769-782.

Sweet, J. A. *Women in the labor force.* New York: Seminar, 1973.

Sweet, J. A. The impact of recent fertility and nuptiality trends on the employment and work experience of young women (CDE Working Paper 79-17). Madison: Center for Demography and Ecology, University of Wisconsin, 1979. (a)

Sweet, J. A. Recent occupational change: How have recent changes in fertility and marriage affected the occupational distribution of young women (CDE Working Paper 79-18). Madison: Center for Demography and Ecology, University of Wisconsin, 1979. (b)

Sweet, J. A. Changes in the amount and sources of income of young married couples: 1960-1976 (CDE Working Paper 79-42). Madison: Center for Demography and Ecology, University of Wisconsin, 1979. (c)

Sweet, J. A. Recent trends in the size and composition of income of young Black couples: 1960-1976 (CDE Working Paper 80-10). Madison: Center for Demography and Ecology, University of Wisconsin, 1980.

Turchi, B. Micro economic theories of fertility: A critique. *Social Forces* 1975, 54(1), 107-125.

Veevers, J. E. Voluntarily childless wives: An exploratory study. *Sociology and Social Research: An International Journal,* 1973, 57(2), 356-366.

Waite, L. J. *Women, work and the family.* Paper presented at the meetings of the American Sociological Association, New York, 1980. (a)

Waite, L. J. Working wives and the family life cycle. *American Journal of Sociology,* 1980, 86(2), 272. (b)

Waite, L. J., and Stolzenberg, R. M. Intended childbearing and labor force participation of young women: Insights from nonrecursive models. *American Journal of Sociology,* 1976, 41, 235-52.

Westoff, C. F., Potter, R. G., Sagi, P. C., and Mishler, E. G. *Family growth in metropolitan America.* Princeton, NJ: Princeton University Press, 1961.

Westoff, C. F., Potter, R. G., and Sagi, P. C. *The third child child.* Princeton, NJ: Princeton University Press, 1963.

Williams, G. The changing U.S. labor force and occupational differentiation by sex. *Demography,* 1979, 16, 73-87.

Willis, R. J. A new approach to the economic theory of fertility behavior. *Journal of Political Economy,* 1973, 81, S14-S64.

Wolf, W. C., and Fligstein, N. Sex and authority in the workplace: Causes of sexual inequality. *American Sociological Review,* 1979, 44(2), 235-252. (a)

Wolf, W. C., and Fligstein, N. Sexual stratification: Differences in power in the work setting. *Social Forces,* 1979, 58, 94-107. (b)

10

Measuring the Impact of Marital Discord, Dissolution, and Remarriage on Fertility

Helen P. Koo and C. M. Suchindran

In assessing the impact of marital dissolution and remarriage on fertility, a number of difficulties must be dealt with. First, there are several issues that must be addressed because of the nature of the problem. Second, the data available for studying the problem have various deficiencies. Third, even working within the limitations of the available data, one must face several pitfalls. Below, we will

WE GRATEFULLY acknowledge the contributions of Andrew Cherlin, Janet D. Griffith, and Arland Thornton, who reviewed the manuscript; Rebecca A. Teeter and Carol A. Martell, who provided programming assistance; and Debra Harris and Elva Deboy, who typed the manuscript and tables. The research was supported by Contract NO1-HD-52838 and Grant RO1-HD-13709 from the Center for Population Research of the National Institute of Child Health and Human Development; the writing of the chapter was partially supported by a Professional Development Award from Research Triangle Institute.

discuss each of these three categories of difficulties in turn, before offering examples of some possible approaches to resolving them. The approaches that we discuss are those we feel to be of more general use or interest; we apply them using retrospective survey data.

GENERAL ISSUES

Regardless of the type of data used to investigate the effects of conjugal experience on childbearing, several points must be kept in mind.

Two-Way Relationship

It is difficult to measure the impact of marital discord, disruption,[1] and remarriage on fertility because the network of relationships among these phenomena is extremely complex. First, the direction of cause and effect extends both ways between childbearing and marital events. Within marriage, in one direction of causality, marital tensions (that eventually result in separation and divorce) may influence couples' decisions to have children — either to avoid having children or any additional ones, or to have a(another) child in hopes of holding their marriage together. In the opposite direction from causality, the fertility of couples may influence the stability of their union, and the effects may also be either positive or negative: The rewards of having children may cement conjugal bonds, but problems of childbearing and childrearing may result in marital stress and dissolution. After the marriage has ended, marital dissolution may influence fertility by removing some of the affected individuals from the sexually active or procreating population for significant periods of time. At a later stage still, the relationship between remarriage and childbearing is again a reciprocal one. Entering into a new marriage may affect a couple's fertility. For example, regardless of the number of children from previous unions, they may bear children to "validate" the new union; or they may choose not to have children to avoid the complications of raising step- or half-siblings. On the other hand, the number and ages of children from previous marriages may influence the likelihood that divorced people remarry.

In assessing the impact of marital discord, dissolution, and remarriage on fertility, one must recognize that even though we wish to focus attention on one direction of the two-way relationship, one must take into account the opposite direction of effects. One way to do this is to estimate a system of simultaneous equations, in which the reciprocal effects are specified and the influence of marital experience on fertility, *net* of the opposite effect (of childbearing on marital history), can be estimated. Few such attempts have been made on this topic, however. Koo and Janowitz (1981) have estimated a simultaneous logit model to study the interrelationships between marital dissolution and fertility around the time of the separation, and they discuss the difficulties of such undertakings. Because so few empirical works have been done in this area, we shall not discuss simultaneous equation systems further in this chapter.

Another approach is to ignore the reciprocal nature of the relationship and simply estimate in an one-way equation the effects of marital events on fertility. Although this has been the most frequently used method (e.g., see Grabill et al., 1958; Lauriat, 1969; Palmore and Ariffin, 1969; Cohen and Sweet, 1974; Thornton, 1978), the results are affected to an unknown degree by simultaneity bias.

Stage of Marriage

Another aspect of the complexity of the interrelationships between marital events and childbearing is that the interrelationships extend over long periods of time, during which the effects may vary. Thus, the impact of discord or remarriage on childbearing may be different at the beginning or middle as opposed to the end of a union. One may deal with this problem by studying the effects by each succeeding year of marriage, or by each successive age, or by focusing attention on the effects in more general stages of marital history. It is important to note that if one does not take into account the stage of marriage being investigated, results may be misleading and not comparable with those of other studies.

Men versus Women

The effects of marital instability and remarriage on fertility may differ for men and women. Because men are much less likely than women to take day-to-day responsibility for children, especially after unions have ended, the impact of marital dissolution or remarriage on men's subsequent childbearing may be less than on women's. Consequently, one should make separate assessments for the two sexes. We will not address this issue further, however, because there are so little data for doing so: Men's reproductive histories (along with marital histories) are rarely available. Therefore, hereafter, we speak of the effects for women only.

Comparison Group

In measuring the effect of marital events on fertility, one needs to consider what women's childbearing histories *would have been* had they *not* undergone marital discord, disruption, or remarriage. To make an appraisal, one ideally would compare women's actual fertility (after having been exposed to discord, disruption, and remarriage) with their "expected" fertility (in the absence of these marital experiences). Because this "expected" fertility is, by its nature, never known; and because substitutes, such as women's reports of what they think they would have done reproductively had their conjugal histories been different, cannot be validated and in any case are not generally available, it is necessary to compare the reproductive performance of women who experience unstable unions and remarriages with that of a comparison group. The fertility of this comparison group is taken to approximate the expected fertility of the maritally disrupted group in the absence of marital instability. The choice of this comparison group is obviously crucial to the outcome of the assessment. As we will see, the fertility of such a comparison group need not be the actual childbearing of a group, but can be a synthetic fertility schedule derived from actual experience.

Secular Change

Rates of fertility, marital dissolution, and remarriage have undergone dramatic changes in recent decades. In evaluating the effects of disruption and remarriage on fertility for women experiencing these phenomena at different historical periods, it is important not to confuse changes in fertility due to secular trends (or other exogenous events) with the reproductive impact made specifically by marital instability. One way to sort out the secular changes from the effects being studied is to control for birth or marriage cohort (women born or married during the same period), and for the time period during which the events occur, so that women who experienced the fertility and marital rates of given periods are (in some sense) studied separately.

Other Confounding Factors

Besides needing to avoid the spurious effects that could be produced by secular trends in vital rates, one must control for the effects of factors other than marital history that affect reproductive behavior. Such characteristics as women's religion, education, and labor force commitment, for example, influence women's childbearing, as well as their matrimonial behavior (propensity to dissolve and reenter unions). Without taking into account the influence of such factors, one could attribute to marital events differences in fertility patterns that are actually due to the other variables.

Loss and Compensation

Another general issue that needs to be dealt with is that not only may couples' childbearing be decreased (or increased) by the experience of conjugal discord and dissolution, the effect may be offset by their fertility during the time they are separated or divorced, and also by their childbearing after remarriage. To assess the "total" effect of marital events on fertility, this compensating mechanism needs to be taken into account.

Specific methods for dealing with some of the problems outlined above will be presented in a later section, after data problems have been discussed.

DATA

Ideal Data

As a way of highlighting the inadequacies that must be overcome in the data available for examining the impact of marital events on reproduction, we first outline the kinds of data that would be ideal. To aid in disentangling the interrelationships among a series of events over time, a *prospective* study on a representative sample of couples married during a given period would collect information over the course of the marriages, from the beginning through their dissolution (if any) and subsequent remarriages (if any). To help elucidate the interrelationships between marital harmony (and discord) and decisions about childbearing, one would collect, at successive time points in a union, each partner's feelings of satisfaction and dissatisfaction about various aspects of the marriage and their attitudes and behavior in resolving conjugal conflicts (including the willingness and ability to resort to dissolution of the union), as well as each spouse's attitudes, motivations, decisions, and outcomes regarding having a child or an additional child during the various periods of time. One would also obtain in successive periods measures of the socioeconomic circumstances of the couple (education, occupation, income and assets, and the like) and of their psychological status (such as personality characteristics, various motivational strengths, and attitudes) so as to be able to control for other factors influencing marital and childbearing behavior.

Available Data

The ideal data described do not exist. There are other data, however, that can be utilized to investigate the effects of marital discord, dissolution, and remarriage on fertility; but their use requires care in specifying the underlying assumptions that allow their utilization and in recognizing the limitations that cannot be overcome.

For assessing the impact of marital events on fertility in a population, the representativeness and size of the sample from which data are collected are crucial.[2] For this reason, in the absence of any *prospective* study on a probability sample that focuses on marital and fertility behavior,[3] we prefer data from *retrospective,* cross-sectional studies based on large probability samples.[4] Retrospective surveys collect (at one point in time) information covering long periods in the past. Below, we discuss some aspects of such retrospective data for the purposes at hand. Later, we describe other kinds of data that may be used for measuring the impact of marital history on fertility.

The minimum requirement that such retrospective survey data must meet to be suitable to the problem at hand is that they contain complete (or nearly complete) fertility and marital histories — that is, the dates of each pregnancy or birth and of the beginning and end of each marriage. Examples of such surveys are the series of national fertility surveys in the U.S., starting in 1955 (the most recent ones being the 1970 National Fertility Survey and the 1973 and 1976 National Survey of Family Growth) and the June supplements to the 1971, 1975, and 1980 Current Population Surveys. Survey data fulfilling these requirements generally do not also include information on marital discord and related data, or on the decision-making process and associated factors regarding childbearing. Consequently, one must use the act of separation or divorce as an indicator of marital discord that existed at an earlier time or times. However, because the genesis of conditions leading to marital dissolution (including marital stress) is often gradual, occurring (sometimes on and off) over long periods of time, one cannot determine from the timing of the dissolution itself the point at which during a given marriage marital strife began affecting childbearing behavior. One must assume that in some cases conjugal dissatisfaction could start influencing fertility from the very beginning of unions, while in most cases, it probably has an effect at least in the period immediately before the dissolution (if reproduction is still possible).

In the case of pregnancies or births, one cannot assume their occurrence to indicate preexisting desire to have a child, since pregnancies may be unwanted accidents. What is of interest here, however, is not how marital events affect fertility *planning,* but *actual fertility.* Thus, the occurrence of pregnancies can be used in measuring the effects of marital instability on childbearing. The use of birth (as opposed to pregnancy) data for this purpose, however, requires the assumption that couples in unstable unions or remarriages are no more likely than others to be subject to fetal loss. While there is no reason to expect any difference in miscarriage or stillbirth rates, it is possible that those experiencing marital instability undergo a somewhat higher incidence of induced abortion.[5]

Given these caveats, one may use data on marital and fertility histories obtained in retrospective surveys to measure the impact of dissolution and remarriage on fertility. There are certain analytical problems that must be resolved in doing so, however. These are discussed in the following section.

Another type of large-scale data is census data. However, the U.S. Bureau of the Census does not obtain marital or fertility histories, but only current marital status and the number of children ever born, along with the birth dates of children residing in the household. Thus, limited micro-level analysis of the relationship of marital experience to inferred childbearing can be done (see Lauriat, 1969).

Vital registration data of marriages and divorces and of births do not contain sufficient data on individuals for micro-level analysis. But macro-level studies of the relationships between the divorce (or remarriage) rates and fertility rates, in either cross-sections or time series, are possible using these data. Census data can also be used for such purposes. Such studies are subject to problems of interpretation (the well-known problem of ecological fallacy), however.

PROBLEMS IN ANALYZING
RETROSPECTIVE SURVEY DATA

Some problems common to analyzing retrospective, cross-sectional survey data need to be addressed before we give specific examples of different approaches to estimating the impact of marital events on fertility.

Respondents in a cross-sectional survey are of different ages at the time of interview, and therefore have had varying durations of marital and reproductive (or any other) experience by that time. For example, women who are young when surveyed have had only a few childbearing years, while women past 45 or 50 have completed the reproductive period. In addition, if one is studying events within first marriages (for example), not only does the survey cut off marital histories at varying durations, but marital disruption also ends marriages after different lengths. It is necessary to take these varying durations into account in analyzing fertility of first marriages. For example, for women who first married in a given year (say 15 years before the survey), those who have dissolved their unions at any time before the survey have had fewer years of marriage than those who have not. Thus, they are likely to have borne fewer children (or to be childless) than women whose unions have remained intact to the time of the survey. Unless this result holds true after the difference in marital duration has been adjusted for — that is, after this "truncation bias" has been taken into account — one cannot conclude that women whose marriages have been disrupted experience lower fertility *because* of the marital strife (and dissolution) rather than simply because of the shorter time spent in the wedded state.

One way to adjust for varying marital durations is to examine events in each successive year of completed experience. This can be accomplished by life table techniques or by constructing duration-specific fertility indices, as in the examples given below. To control for the influence of secular trends and other factors, both methods could be performed for subgroups formed by cross-classification of the relevant variables, such as marriage cohorts (for secular trends) by age at marriage by education. To do this in reality is difficult, however, because of the large number of cases that would be required. For this reason, in our basic examples of these techniques, we control for few (if any) factors. In a further example, we illustrate how effects of other variables may be taken into account by performing multivariate analysis of life tables.

COMPARISON GROUPS AND CONFOUNDING FACTORS

In this and subsequent sections, we illustrate some approaches to the problems discussed earlier. These examples are chosen to illustrate the methodological issues raised, rather than to present empirical evidence for substantive conclusions. Such conclusions should not be drawn from the results presented here because the examples given are not complete works. Furthermore, it is important to note that in all of our examples of estimating the impact of marital events on fertility, the reverse relationship has not been taken into account. Therefore, as discussed earlier, the results are affected by simultaneity bias, the direction and extent of which are unknown. Below we examine ways to handle the selected issues in turn.

Previous works investigating the effects of marital strife, dissolution, and remarriage on fertility have compared the childbearing of women whose first marriages were intact at the time of interview with that of women who have dissolved their unions and/or who have remarried by the time of interview, controlling for various factors (Lauriat, 1969; Cohen and Sweet, 1974; Thornton, 1978). They have attributed differences in the fertility of the two groups to the effects of marital disruption, remarriage, and, in some cases, the conjugal conflict suffered before the dissolution. Thus, they have assumed that the reproductive experience of the women in intact marriages represents the fertility that the women who have terminated their unions and/or remarried would have experienced had they not undergone marital discord, disruption, or remarriage.

Two problems trouble this approach. First, women whose marriages are still intact at interview may end their unions at some time after the survey. (That is, their marital histories are incomplete, having been arbitrarily truncated by the survey, as previously discussed.) Therefore, the women in the intact unions being used as a comparison group do not represent a "true" stably married group;

some of them have also experienced or will experience marital discord and will eventually separate and divorce.

The second problem is that even among women who truly remain stably married (that is, who will never voluntarily terminate their unions after the survey), some have undergone conjugal distress during their childbearing years but, for a variety of reasons, have never ended their unions.

As we shall see, for purposes of estimating the impact of marital discord on childbearing during marriage, the problems (without direct data on marital discord) are, to a degree, intractable. But one can calculate effects that to some extent either underestimate or overestimate the impact. To this point we will return in the examples below. But for purposes of estimating the impact of conjugal strife on fertility during a specific period, namely, near the end of the union, and for assessing the effects of marital disruption itself (that is, via removal of women from exposure to the risk of pregnancy) or of remarriage on fertility, the problems can be at least partially resolved. Our suggested solution is to use a group other than women in intact first marriages at the time of survey as a comparison group. This approach is illustrated in subsequent sections.

Below we illustrate some ways to explore the extent to which these problems combined may affect the measurement of the impact of marital discord on childbearing.

Cumulative Fertility Rates

Using data from the 1973 National Survey of Family Growth, which contains women aged 15 to 44 at the time of survey, we constructed a schedule of marital duration-specific fertility rates expected for women still in first marriages when interviewed if their fertility histories had not been censored by the survey. This was done by calculating for successive six-month periods of marriage the birth rates for women in intact marriages who had been married that long, and then cumulating the rates to generate duration-specific cumulated fertility rates. Premarital births were added to month 0 of marriage and included in the cumulation. The results are presented for selected durations in columns 1 and 4 of Table 10.1 for black and white women who married at age 20 or older.

A similar schedule was constructed for women whose first marriages had been dissolved by the time of the survey. In each duration, only women whose unions had remained intact to that time were

TABLE 10.1 Mean Numbers of Births Expected for Women First Married at Age 20 or Older

Time Since First Marriage Began	Blacks						Whites					
	Intact First Marriage (1)		Ever Separated From First Marriage				Intact First Marriage (4)		Ever Separated From First Marriage			
			Fertility in First Marriage (2)		Fertility in All Marriages (3)				Fertility in First Marriage (5)		Fertility in All Marriages (6)	
	Rate	S.E.	Rate	S.E.	Rate	S.E.	Rate	S.E.	Rate	S.E.	Rate	S.E.
0 Months	.62	.04	.85	.06	.85	.06	.05	.01	.14	.02	.14	.02
6 Months	.75	.04	.98	.06	.98	.06	.09	.01	.18	.03	.18	.03
1 Year	.97	.05	1.25	.07	1.20	.06	.30	.01	.42	.04	.43	.04
2	1.28	.05	1.58	.07	1.50	.07	.61	.02	.74	.05	.73	.05
3	1.54	.06	1.85	.08	1.74	.07	.92	.02	.96	.06	.91	.05
4	1.76	.06	2.09	.08	1.96	.08	1.22	.02	1.26	.07	1.15	.06
5	1.98	.06	2.27	.09	2.04	.08	1.48	.03	1.56	.08	1.36	.07
10	2.78	.07	2.89	.12	2.71	.09	2.27	.03	2.28	.12	1.94	.08
15	3.22	.09	3.21	.16	2.98	.10	2.60	.04	2.49	.13	2.21	.10
20 Years	3.47	.10	3.21	.16	3.12	.11	2.67	.04	2.56	.15	2.29	.10

Data: 1973 National Survey of Family Growth.

included in the calculation. Thus, these cumulative fertility rates represent the number of children expected to be born by given marital durations to women who underwent marital dissolution if they had *not* terminated their unions but had remained married (presumably in the presence of conjugal strife that preceded the disruption) and had gone on to experience the fertility rates of women whose marriages lasted longer. These results are seen in columns 2 and 5 of Table 10.1.

Comparing the two marital groups, one sees that for both races, the disrupted group had a higher rate of premarital births (month 0) than the intact group (p < .05 for whites, .05 < p < .10 for blacks). If births conceived before marriage (that is, births occurring by 0 and 6 months of marriage) are subtracted from the cumulative rate for the twentieth year, the result represents the cumulative rate of fertility occurring within marriage. This cumulative "marital" fertility rate of the disrupted group was lower than that of the intact group for both races, but the difference was significant only for blacks (p < .01).[6]

Differences in the timing of fertility within marriage are also apparent. For example, among women marrying at 20 or older, blacks in the intact group had half of their expected cumulative marital fertility by 5.62 years, whereas those in the disrupted group took 4.06 years. The corresponding figures for whites were 4.62 and 4.37 years.

These results indicate that, for some subgroups at least, the fertility of the disrupted group expected *in the absence of dissolution but in the presumed presence of marital discord* differed from that of the intact group. Although the intact group contains some women who will end their marriages in the future as well as others who have experienced conjugal strife but who will never separate or divorce, one could assume that the proportion of women in this group who suffered marital disharmony (that could have influenced their fertility) would be smaller than the proportion (presumably 100 percent) in the disrupted group.

Then, everything else equal, the difference in marital fertility of the two groups could be attributed to the effects of the greater conjugal discord influencing the expected childbearing of the disrupted group. (In this example, one should not assume everything else *is* equal, especially since we have not controlled for a number of possibly relevant factors.)

Now, if we make the assumption that the fertility of those women in the intact group who will dissolve their unions in the future (and also that the fertility of those women in this group who suffer conjugal conflict but who never separate) is the same as that of the women already in the disrupted group, then the estimated expected fertility of the disrupted group is not biased. But the expected fertility of the intact group *is* biased to the extent that marital discord influences childbearing there.

Under this assumption, if the estimated expected fertility of the disrupted group is significantly *lower* than that of the intact group (as in the case of blacks married at 20 or older), then the overall effect of discord is to depress fertility, and thus the estimated expected fertility of the intact group underestimates the fertility of the "true" intact group (because of the presence of discord-affected women). Consequently, the difference in expected fertility between the disrupted and intact group is also underestimated, and the "true" difference would be larger and also, therefore, significant.

If the expected fertility of the disrupted group is significantly *greater* than that of the intact group (as in the case of blacks married at less than 20), then, overall, discord raises fertility. Following the same reasoning as in the previous case, we see that the estimated difference in expected fertility between the two groups is also underestimated, and the "true" difference would be larger and also significant. Thus, in both cases, the estimates are conservative ones, and one can safely infer from the estimated difference that discord has an effect on fertility (in the direction observed).

However, if the estimated expected fertility of the two groups is *not* significantly different (as in the case of white women), then no conclusions can be drawn. The true situation could be that there is no difference, or that there actually is a difference in either direction.

In summary, the results presented indicate that among black women who married at young ages, marital discord increased marital fertility, while among blacks marrying at average or older ages, it had the opposite effect. Among whites, however, no inferences can be made. Below we further explore the question for white women, using different (though related) techniques and different data.

Life Table Techniques

The method of using the parts of fertility histories that were completed before the survey or before marital dissolution in order to compute expected cumulative fertility rates over time effectively eliminates truncation bias. Life table techniques are based on the same principle (see Sheps, 1965). Life table methods offer advantages over the other method, however: (1) Whereas the experience of women who do not complete a given interval (for instance, those who are cut off by the survey during year 5) is ignored in the previous method (omitted from the fifth-year computation), life table techniques incorporate their experience into the interval. The disadvantage of omitting such women becomes particularly serious when large intervals must be used. (2) The probabilities of experiencing a *series* of events (such as births and/or marriages of successive orders) rather than just one event may be examined and encapsulated in summary indices in a certain kind of life table (increment-decrement life tables; see Suchindran et al., 1977). (3) Life table rates are amenable to multivariate analysis by means of Cox models or proportional hazards models (Cox, 1972), or by categorical data analysis (Koch et al., 1972). Below we illustrate, in turn, the use of ordinary or multiple-decrement life tables, increment-decrement life tables, and Cox models. In these examples, we further study the possible effects of marital discord on first-marriage fertility.

Multiple-Decrement Life Tables

To study fertility, one may examine not only the number of children born but the length of time elapsed between marriage and first birth, and between successive births (birth intervals), or the probabilities over time of attaining each parity. With life table techniques, in studying the probability or timing of birth n (say, the second birth), the experiences of women who have had the prior birth n − 1 (first birth), but have not yet had birth n by the time of the survey or of marital disruption, are included in the calculations, thus avoiding truncation bias.

To illustrate these techniques, we compare the birth intervals within first marriages of women classified by whether they have experienced disruption of their first unions. However, rather than simply grouping together all women who ever dissolved their first marriages, for this example we further divided this group into three categories, according to women's marital experience up to the time of the survey: women separated or divorced from first marriage (MD), those remarried after a first divorce (MDM), and those twice divorced (MDMD).[7] We made this further distinction because we wished to explore the possibility that women with differing marital experiences were characterized by different fertility patterns. Of course, the same truncation problem exists here: the women in the M (intact first marriages), MD, and MDM groups may experience a marital dissolution or remarriage subsequent to the survey.

We used data for white women from the June 1975 Current Population Survey, because its large sample size provides sufficient cases of the more complex marital patterns for analysis. Women who experienced premarital births were excluded from the life table analysis because of difficulty in determining the exposure time for births. Also, lack of cases, especially in the MD and MDMD patterns, prohibited calculation of separate life tables for age-at-marriage groups. Women with multiple births were also excluded because of difficulty in defining the length of the order-specific birth intervals.

We constructed multiple-decrement life tables treating births of a specific order and separation or divorce (or withdrawals due to survey cutoff date) as decrements for each marital pattern. From these life tables, associated single-decrement life tables were constructed treating birth of a specific order as the only risk, thus eliminating the effect of separation or divorce (or withdrawals due to survey cutoff date) on reproductive performance. The life table probabilities over time of having a birth of a specific order were used to compare fertility across marital patterns. We tested the significance of differences among these probability curves by using the Peto and Pykes test (see Suchindran and Lingner, 1977). The life table also provides summary measures such as parity progression ratios, which measure the level of fertility, and median birth intervals, which measure the spacing of children.

Table 10.2 presents the life table probabilities of having a first birth by given durations of first marriage in the absence of disruption or withdrawal due to the survey cutoff date for the four marital groups. The median first-order birth intervals computed from these survival probabilities were 1.71, 1.46, 1.57, and 1.70 years, respectively, for the M, MD, MDM, and MDMD groups. The parity progression ratios (which in this case are the probabilities having a birth in 20 years) were .9061, .8813, .8756, and 9037, respectively, for the four marital patterns. No significant differences were found in the probability distributions of the four marital groups ($x^2 = 2.34$, df = 3, p > .05).

Similar life tables were constructed for the second through fifth birth intervals (see Koo and Suchindran, 1978). There were no significant differences in the probability distributions over time of having the first three births among the four groups, but the distributions were

TABLE 10.2   Life Table Cumulative Probabilities of a First Birth (white women with no premarital births)

Duration of First Marriage in Years	Marital Group[a]			
	M	MD	MDM	MDMD
0	.2605	.3190	.2887	.3112
1	.5328	.5815	.5503	.5977
2	.6668	.6898	.6700	.7042
3	.7456	.7479	.7249	.7531
4	.7979	.7816	.7674	.7778
5	.8312	.8109	.7910	.8154
6	.8511	.8233	.8087	.8412
7	.8662	.8302	.8204	.8692
8	.8761	.8424	.8372	.8797
9	.8831	.8485	.8430	.8797
10	.8891	.8554	.8499	.8797
20	.9061	.8813	.8756	.9037
Median birth interval (in years)[b]	1.71	1.46	1.57	1.70
Sample size	21,302	2,172	1,959	338

Data: June 1975 Current Population Survey.

a. See text for definition.

b. Duration by which 50 percent of women had a first birth, among those who had a first birth in 20 years.

significantly different among the four groups in the fourth and fifth birth intervals. In these higher birth orders, currently divorced women (MD and MDMD) had significantly higher parity progression ratios and shorter median birth intervals than currently married women (M and MDM).

Because membership in the four marital groups may change after the survey and because some women in a given group may nevertheless share the unmeasured factors influencing women in another group, the life table estimates above are subject to biases similar to those discussed in the section on cumulative fertility rates. Following the same reasoning (and under the same assumptions as before) to assess the direction of bias, we again can conclude that if significant differences are found, then the "true" differences are actually larger and therefore also significant, and effects in the direction estimated can be inferred; but if the estimated differences are not significant, then the direction of the bias is not certain and no conclusions can be

TABLE 10.3   Mean Numbers of Births Expected in the Absence of
Marital Dissolution (white women with no premarital
births)[a]

Duration of First Marriage in Years	Marital Group[b]			
	M	*MD*	*MDM*	*MDMD*
1	0.26	0.31	0.29	0.31
2	0.57	0.64	0.61	0.67
3	0.86	0.93	0.86	0.92
4	1.12	1.16	1.11	1.12
5	1.37	1.38	1.31	1.36
10	2.18	2.15	1.97	2.17
20	2.67	2.77	2.45	2.65

Data: June 1975 Current Population Survey.

a. Calculated from increment-decrement life table.

b. See text for definition.

drawn. (These considerations apply to the example below as well, and will not be repeated there.)

Consequently, the results in this example indicate that marital discord and other factors related to marital behavior increased the first-marriage fertility of white women who had dissolved their first and second unions and who at the time of the survey had not married again, by increasing their probabilities of having higher-order births.

Increment-Decrement
Life Tables

Life table techniques can be used also to study *cumulative* fertility. Increment-decrement life tables give a complete picture of family-building by incorporating all parities into one table, as opposed to multiple-decrement life tables, which require a separate table for each birth order. The former type of life tables provides summary measures such as average number of children expected to be born in the absence of separation or divorce but in the presence of presumed preceding marital stress (or in the absence of withdrawal due to survey cutoff date) in a given duration of first marriage.

Using the same data as in the previous example, we constructed such a life table; results are presented in Table 10.3. The expected completed fertility (that is, the number of children at the end of the twentieth year of first marriage in the absence of disruption or survey cutoff) was lowest for MDM women and highest for MD women.

This is consistent with the multiple-decrement life table results. The number of children expected by duration of first marriage shows that M women had fewer births in the first two years of marriage but caught up with the other groups by the beginning of year 5. Although the M D group experienced a slight dip in the tenth year of marriage, in general they had a high average number of children at all marital durations.

Multivariate Analysis
of Life Tables

In the life table examples above, the influence of other factors on fertility was not taken into account. Here we illustrate a multivariate method of analyzing probabilities produced by multiple-decrement life tables that adjusts statistically for the effects of other variables. Unlike other regression techniques, this method, known as proportional hazards or Cox models, makes use of the incomplete (censored) data and thus controls for truncation bias (for details, see Cox, 1972; Kalbfleish and Prentice, 1980).

To illustrate this method, we reexamine the probabilities of having a first birth in the marriage for women who at the time of survey were in intact first marriages and for those who had at some time experienced disruption of the first union, controlling for the influence of age at marriage, education, and birth cohort. This exercise explores multivariately the problem presented above in the section illustrating multiple-decrement life tables, except that for simplicity, we group together the women who ever experienced disruption of a first marriage.

The results are presented in Table 10.4. In contrast to the outcome that the differences in the probability of first birth among the marital groups was not significant in Table 10.2, here the difference was highly significant when the effects of the other factors were taken into account. The intact group was significantly more likely to have a first birth than the disrupted group (in the absence of separation or divorce). As discussed earlier, the size of the difference, presumed to be due to marital discord, is underestimated.

As seen in Table 10.4, all coefficients of all categories of all variables were significant at the .10 level. The probability of having a first birth decreased with each category of age at marriage. The coefficient for the oldest (omitted) category is computed by summing the negatives of the coefficients of the included categories, or −0.411.

TABLE 10.4 Estimated Regression Coefficients in Cox Model of Probability of First Birth (white women with no premarital births)

Variable[a]	Estimated Coefficients[b]	Standard Error	P value
Age at First Marriage			
Less than 18	.3393	.0151	<.0001
18-20	.1553	.0113	<.0001
21-24	−.0833	.0124	<.0001
Education			
Less than 9 years	.0478	.0249	.0554
9-11	.0292	.0165	.0770
12	.0712	.0249	.0043
Birth Cohort			
1900-1914	−.2360	.0171	<.0001
1915-1929	.0199	.0120	.0964
1930-1944	.2337	.0116	<.0001
Marital Group			
Intact first marriage vs. ever separated	.0441	.0100	<.0001

Data: June 1975 Current Population Survey.

a. The omitted categories for Age at First Marriage, Education, and Birth Cohorts are "Age 25+", "More than 12 years of schooling," and "Born after 1944" respectively.

b. The coefficients are estimated as deviations from the overall mean rather than from the omitted category.

The relative risk of having a first birth for women married at age 17 or younger compared to women married at 25 or older is e^{1339}/e^{51411} or 2.119. That is, women in the youngest age-at-marriage class were twice as likely to have a first birth as those in the oldest category.

The effects of education were not monotonic. Women who completed twelve years of school had the highest probability of a first birth, while those with at least some college had the lowest.

As is evident in Table 10.4, the coefficients for birth cohorts reflect the well-known changes in birth rates during the Great Depression, the postwar baby boom, and the subsequent low-fertility period.

In summary, the effects of marital experience were not significant when examined by the multiple-decrement life tables which did not control for other factors, but were significant when other variables were taken into account in the Cox model. This exercise demonstrates the importance of adjusting for the influence of confounding factors, including cohort-period effects.

Other multivariate methods may also be used to study the impact of discord on fertility, including multiple classification analysis, ordinary least squares, logit, and probit techniques. These methods do not analyze life table probabilities, however, so care must be taken to avoid the effects of truncation bias. One way to do this is to include in a particular analysis only women who have had at least a given duration of experience (see Becker et al., 1977; Thornton, 1977). Another method that has been used (for example, by Cohen and Sweet, 1974) is to control for duration by including it explicitly as an independent variable in the equation. When the data contain a cross-section of women of different ages, however, the maximum duration measured for any given woman is determined by the time of interview; thus, the measured duration is not the "true" duration, and the result of including duration as an independent variable is that the estimates of all coefficients tend to be biased and inconsistent (see Koo and Suchindran, 1980).

In addition, it is also possible to control for the effects of several factors simultaneously by standardizing fertility rates on a number of variables (for example, see Thornton, 1978).

STAGE OF MARRIAGE

It was noted earlier that the effects of marital experience on fertility may be different at different stages of marriage. In this section, we discuss some ways of examining this question within first marriage. A later section studies this problem with respect to periods following the end of first marriage.

Successive Periods of Marriage

One way to examine whether effects of marital discord on childbearing behavior vary over the course of marriage is to compare the successive duration-specific fertility rates of the intact and disrupted groups. These marital duration-specific rates were cumulated to form the cumulative rates presented in columns 1, 2, 4, and 5 of Table 10.1 (discussed previously). Because we wished to study the effects of discord on childbearing within marriage, we compared the duration-specific fertility rates starting with year 1, excluding premarital births and premaritally conceived births. To smooth over the random fluctuations in the six-month rates, we computed rates for two-year durations.

For each two-year marital duration, we calculated the ratio of the intact group's fertility rate to that of the disrupted group and tested for statistical significance. Earlier we had shown that the expected average number of children born within marriage among blacks married at age 20 or older was significantly lower for the disrupted than for the intact group. When we examined the ratios, we found that in years 1-2, the expected fertility rate of the disrupted group was significantly higher than that of the intact group. In subsequent years, the disrupted group's expected fertility was lower, but the difference was not significant until years 9-10 and later.

Similarly, among whites wed at 20 or older, the total marital fertility of the two groups was earlier found not to differ significantly. An examination of the ratios, however, revealed a somewhat different picture. Although the disrupted group's expected fertility rate was higher in years 1-2, the difference was not significant. From years 3-4 onward, the disrupted group had lower fertility. However, this difference was not found to be statistically significant until years 13-14 onward.

In summary, the expected fertility of women who eventually experience marital dissolution may differ significantly from that of other women in some years of marriage and not others, but their expected total fertility within marriage may or may not be different. Thus, it is important to investigate the effects of marital discord on childbearing at different points in time within marriage.[8]

Period Around the End of Marriage

Thornton (1978) has suggested that marital discord resulting in separation may be concentrated in the period immediately preceding the dissolution. He therefore compared the fertility of women who had ever separated from their first unions during the period spanning 18 months prior to separation to 6 months following it, to the childbearing of women in intact first marriages during a corresponding time period. As discussed earlier, the use of women in intact unions as a comparison group biases the results, because some of these women will separate after the survey and others who will not do so nevertheless have suffered conjugal conflict. In addition, even if the effects of a number of other variables are controlled for, the two groups inevitably differ in many other characteristics. If there is reason to believe that the assumption is valid that marital discord does not substantially affect fertility until a given period before separation, we can for the most part eliminate these problems by selecting as the comparison group a subgroup of the women in the disrupted group.

Specifically, we suggest that the average number of children born during the chosen period prior to dissolution (for example, 18 months prior to separation to 6 months afterwards) be computed for women who have ever separated from the first marrriage and classified by durations since the wedding when the disruption occurred. For each such category of women by time when separation occurred, the comparison group would be women who separated subsequent to the end of this period — in this case, 24 or more months later. The fertility of each comparison group during the chosen (24-month) period (that is, during a period when it has been assumed that marital discord has not yet begun for them) would then be compared to that of women who *did* terminate their union (and thus experienced discord) during this period. The primary advantage of using this method is that the comparison group represents a subgroup of the disrupted group who happened to have dissolved their unions later. Therefore, they would not be expected to differ in many characteristics, reducing the need to control for the effects of confounding variables.

This procedure, however, would yield estimates that are accurate only to the extent that the assumption is valid that conjugal strife affects childbearing only during the chosen period preceding the dissolution. If the assumption is substantially violated — if discord significantly influences fertility either consistently or sporadically throughout marriage — then the previously discussed method of examining cumulative fertility in successive years of marriage would be more appropriate.

LOSS AND COMPENSATION

We turn our attention now to the decrease in postmarital fertility attributable to the loss of reproductive time experienced by women who become separated and divorced, and to the counterbalancing of any such loss by reproduction while separated or divorced (intermarital births) or during remarriage.

The difference between the actual fertility in first marriages of women who have dissolved their first unions and their expected fertility if their marriages had not ended may be considered to be the "gross loss" in fertility due to the disruption of first unions. This gross loss represents a theoretical concept because, in reality, women go on to reproduce after ending their unions, by producing births while separated or divorced or, if they remarry, by having children in subsequent marriages. If these postdissolution births are subtracted from the gross loss, the result represents the "net loss," that is, the "loss" in fertility net of the compensation through intermarital and remarriage childbearing.

In the section below, we provide an example of how this net loss may be computed. In the following section, we decompose the net loss into the two components, one involving intermarital births and the other, remarriage fertility.

Estimation of Net Loss

The fertility of the disrupted group had they *not* dissolved their unions can be estimated by calculating marital duration-specific cumulated fertility rates using birth rates during periods preceding disruption. This was done previously and presented in columns 2 and 5 of Table 10.1. Such a fertility schedule represents the childbearing expected in the absence of dissolution, and it is this expected experience that should be compared to the actual fertility of the women who have separated, divorced, or remarried to compute the net loss. By using the expected fertility of the *same* women had they not experienced disruption as the comparison schedule, we reduce the need to control for confounding factors. In the past, the fertility of the women who never disrupted their first marriages (seen in columns 1 and 4 of Table 10.1) has been used as the comparison schedule (Lauriat, 1969; Cohen and Sweet, 1974; Thornton, 1978); but as discussed earlier, this practice may bias the results.

The mean number of children that women who ended their first marriages actually had by successive years since the first wedding, including all children born during separation or divorce and in all subsequent unions, are presented in columns 3 and 6 of Table 10.1. In the examples given in Table 10.1, the net loss (at the end of 20 years after beginning first marriage) differs according to whether the expected fertility of the disrupted group (columns 2 or 5) or of the intact group (columns 1 or 4) are compared to the actual fertility. Among blacks and whites marrying at age 20 or older, the net losses of .09 and .27, respectively, computed by subtracting 20-year values in columns 3 and 6 from those in columns 2 and 5, are not significantly different from 0. In contrast, when the 20-year values in columns 1 and 4 are used instead, the net losses (of .35 and .38, respectively) are significantly different from 0. Therefore, one would conclude that there is no significant net loss of fertility due to marital disruption when one utilizes the disrupted group as its own comparison group, whereas one would infer a significant reduction in fertility when one uses the intact group as the comparison group.[9]

Components of Net Loss

The net loss in fertility due to disruption of first marriages may be defined as in the formula below. (The formula may be easily extended to include dissolution of several marriage orders.)

$$\text{Net Loss} = (IM^* - IM) + (R^* - R)$$

Where: IM^* = fertility expected during the period from separation until remarriage or until the end of the reproductive period (whichever comes first) if women had not dissolved the first marriage.

IM = actual fertility while separated or divorced.

R^* = fertility expected during the period from remarriage to the end of the reproductive period if the women had not dissolved the first marriage.

R = actual fertility during remarriage of women who remarried.

The first term represents the part of the net loss due to the difference between women's intermarital births and the fertility they would have had during the corresponding intermarital period, had their marriages not ended. This quantity would be of special interest for examining the implications of changes in intermarital childbearing behavior for the net loss in fertility due to marital disruption. Similarly, the second term, representing the part of the net loss due to the difference in remarriage reproduction and the expected fertility during a corresponding period in the absence of disruption, is of particular interest for examining the implications of changes in remarriage rates and in remarriage fertility for compensating for lost fertility.

A procedure for estimating the first term, $(IM^* - IM)$, has been given in Suchindran and Koo (1980). When survey data containing incomplete marital and fertility histories are used for calculating this quantity, we must be careful to estimate the actual and expected number of intermarital births as well as the length of the period spent

in the separated and divorced status using methods that avoid truncation bias. For this reason, we adopted a method devised by Potter
(1969) utilizing life tables to estimate births averted by contraceptive
use. In our application, marital dissolution is the "contraceptive" and
births while separated or divorced are the "accidental pregnancies."
Again, we prefer the expected fertility of the disrupted group in the
absence of dissolution as the comparison fertility schedule, rather
than the fertility of the intact group.

A simple method for calculating the second term of net loss,
$(R^* - R)$, is outlined here. To estimate R^* (fertility expected during
the remarriage period if women had not ended the first marriage), we
first compute the cumulative fertility rates in each marital duration
expected in the absence of dissolution and remarriage, as in columns 2
and 5 of Table 10.1, under the same assumptions as stated earlier. To
calculate R^*, we obtain for each woman who remarried the fertility
expected during the remarriage period if she had remained in the first
marriage, by taking the difference between the cumulative number of
children born by 20 years and the cumulative number at the time
(since first marriage began) when remarriage occurred. (For example,
as seen in column 2 of Table 10.1, for a black woman who remarried 10
years after her first wedding, the expected fertility is 3.21 − 2.89, or
0.32 children.) R^* is then the mean of these expected numbers of
children for all remarried women.

The calculation of R (actual remarriage fertility) from survey data
with incomplete marital and fertility histories requires the estimation
of the fertility expected during remarriage if histories were completed. This can be done by computing expected second-marriage
cumulative fertility rates by duration since second marriage began, in
a manner analogous to that used for columns 1 and 4 of Table 10.1.
Again, because reproduction in remarriages depends to a large extent
on the age of the woman at remarriage, we would compute the
expected cumulative fertility schedules separately for age at remarriage subgroups. The value of R is obtained by calculating the weighted average of the cumulative fertility at the end of the schedule (say
20 years since remarriage) for the various age-at-remarriage
subgroups.

If there are few data for women with remarriages of long durations, the expected completed fertility would be difficult to estimate.
In this case, it may be possible to utilize information on remarried
women's responses to questions about future additional childbearing.

CONCLUSION

Although many problems confront the enterprise of assessing the impact of marital discord, dissolution, and remarriage on fertility, there are also many ways of overcoming them. We have illustrated some of these methods using data from one-time retrospective surveys. Thus, we have chosen methods that can properly make use of the incomplete histories obtained in such surveys. The techniques that we have illustrated can also be applied to other kinds of data containing incomplete histories, such as panel studies and census data.

At a time when rates of fertility, divorce, and remarriage are all changing rapidly, it is important that we reach a better understanding of how and to what extent marital discord and disruption, and the formation of subsequent unions, influence childbearing behavior. The lack of information on such variables as marital discord and satisfaction, and fertility goals at various points in marriage, limits our ability to address these questions. Thus, more detailed data focusing on these issues need to be collected. In addition, the existing techniques of analysis, such as those we have discussed, should be improved, and alternative methods need to be developed.

NOTES

1. In this chapter we focus attention on marital dissolution due to disaffection rather than death; consequently, the terms "dissolution" and "disruption" are used to mean separation and divorce. Compared to separation and divorce, marital disruption by death has relatively little effect on fertility, because it generally occurs after the prime childbearing years. In addition, it is possible that factors affecting fertility behavior during separation or divorce, or remarriage following divorce, may differ from those influencing reproduction during widowhood or subsequent remarriage. Nevertheless, apart from the sections concerning marital discord, much of the discussion applies to widowhood as well as voluntary marital dissolution.

2. For understanding the mechanisms or processes by which marital events influence childbearing, intensive interview or clinical data from small, nonrepresentative samples may be more useful.

3. To our knowledge, there has been no panel study that has collected both detailed marital and fertility information. There are panel surveys in which some partial marital and fertility or household composition data have been obtained, however, such as the National Longitudinal Survey of the of young and mature men and women (Parnes data), the (national) Panel Study of Income Dynamics, and the National Longitudinal Survey of the high school class of 1972.

4. Retrospective data, however, are subject to more severe recall error than are prospective data.

5. This possibility cannot be evaluated because of the lack of data. However, many women separate while in early pregnancy, and go on to have the child (4 percent of whites and 5 percent of blacks in the 1973 National Survey of Family Growth who had separated from their first husbands were three or fewer months pregnant at the time of separation but carried their pregnancies to term); thus it is possible that once married, even in the face of uncertainty about the continuation of the union, women tend to avoid resorting to induced abortions.

6. A similar table (not presented), constructed for women married at age 19, or younger, showed that this cumulative "marital" fertility rate of women in disrupted marriages was higher rather than lower than that of the intact group. Again, the difference was significant only for blacks ($p < .05$).

7. We did not include more complex histories because of data limitations.

8. However, the effects of simultaneity bias may be especially troublesome in examining fertility rates during successive periods of marriage, and one must be especially cautious in interpreting the results. If the reverse relationship, the impact of childbearing on marital discord (and thus membership in the disrupted group), is not uniform in magnitude or direction throughout various durations of marriage, then the observed differences in duration-specific fertility rates (between the disrupted and the intact groups) through time cannot be simply attributed to marital discord.

9. The results again differ for women marrying at 19 or younger. Among blacks, the net loss was significant when actual fertility was compared to the expected fertility of the disrupted group, but not significant when the fertility of the intact group was used. Among whites, the reduction was not statistically significant with either comparison.

REFERENCES

Becker, G. S., Landes, E. M., and Michael, R. T. An economic analysis of marital instability. *Journal of Political Economy,* 1977 85(6), 1141-1155.

Cohen, S. B., and Sweet, J. A. The impact of marital disruption and remarriage on fertility. *Journal of Marriage and the Family,* 1974 36(1), 87-96.

Cox, D. R. Regression models and life tables (with discussion). *Journal of the Royal Statistical Society,* 1972, B(34), 187-220.

Grabill, W. H., Kiser, C. V., and Whelpton, P. K. *The fertility of American women.* New York: Wiley, 1958.

Kalbfleisch, J. D., and Prentice, R. L. *The statistical analysis of failure time data.* New York: Wiley, 1980.

Koch, G. G., Johnson, W. D., and Tolley, D. A linear model's approach to the analysis of survival and extent of disease in multi-dimensional contingency tables. *Journal of the American Statistical Association,* 1972, 67, 783-796.

Koo, H. P., and Janowitz, B. Effects of childbearing on marital dissolution: Results from a simultaneous logit model. Research Triangle Park, NC: Research Triangle Institute, 1981.

Koo, H. P., and Suchindran, C. M. *Relationships among fertility, marital dissolution, and remarriage.* Final report submitted to the National Institute of Child Health and Human Development, Research Triangle Institute, North Carolina, 1978.

Koo, H. P., and Suchindran, C. M. Effects of children on women's remarriage prospects. *Journal of Family Issues*, 1980, 1(4), 497-515.

Lauriat, P. The effect of marital dissolution on fertility. *Journal of Marriage and the Family*, 1969, 31, 484-493.

Palmore, J. A., and B. M. Ariffin. Marriage patterns and cumulative fertility in West Malaysia, 1966-67. *Demography*, 1969, 6, 383-401.

Potter, R. G. Estimating births averted in a family planning program. In S. J. Behrman et al. (Eds.), *Fertility and family planning: A world view.* Ann Arbor: University of Michigan Press, 1969, 413-434.

Sheps, M. C. An analysis of reproductive patterns in an American isolate. *Population Studies*, 1965, 19, 65-80

Suchindran, C. M., and Koo, H. P. *Divorce, remarriage and fertility.* Paper presented at the annual meeting of the Population Association of America, Denver, April, 1980.

Suchindran, C. M., and Lingner, J. W. On comparison of birth interval distributions. *Journal of Bio-Social Sciences*, 1977, 9, 25-32.

Suchindran, C. M., Namboodiri, N. K., and West, K. Analysis of fertility by increment-decrement life tables. *Proceedings of the American Statistical Association Social Statistics Sections*, 1977, 431-436.

Thornton, A. Children and marital stability. *Journal of Marriage and the Family*, 1977, 39(3), 531-540.

Thornton, A. Marital dissolutions, remarriage, and childbearing. *Demography*, 1978, 15(3), 361-380.

11

Pregnancy Resolution Decisions

A REVIEW AND APPRAISAL OF RESEARCH

Raye Hudson Rosen

While the theme of this book is decision-making, most research in the area of pregnancy resolution has not actually dealt with that process but has tended to focus on correlates of the various pregnancy outcomes: abortion, delivery and releasing of the child for adoption, delivery and keeping the child.[1] Consequently, it is necessary to consider such research, as well as the more recent studies that have begun to examine the processes by which a choice is made. A summary of findings is not the aim here, however. Rather, I am concerned with assessing the direction and quality of this research. Another body of literature, which has been concerned only with the sequelae of pregnancy outcomes, is for the most part outside the scope of this chapter. Since studies that have looked at the male impregnator in relation to pregnancy resolutions have been dealt with in another chapter of this volume, the focus here will be on the bulk of research examining the pregnant female. Two major types of difficulty from which such research has suffered are discussed: (1) problems of theoretical approach, and (2) methodological problems.

THEORETICAL PERSPECTIVES

As has been true of fertility research generally, much work in the area of pregnancy resolution decisions has lacked any articulated theoretical focus and has been concerned primarily with searching out sociodemographic and attitudinal correlates of the various pregnancy resolution decisions (Butts and Sporakowski, 1974; Cushner et al., 1973; Evans et al., 1976; Pakter et al., 1973; Zelnick et al., 1981). This sometimes has been explained as springing from the general lack of knowledge about bases for pregnancy resolutions and a resulting need for exploratory research. For example, Kantner and Zelnick, who have conducted two nationwide surveys of adolescent females 15 through 19 years old, felt it was important at this stage of knowledge to cast a "wide empirical net" (Zelnick et al., 1981: 12). One of their more important findings was the impact of the Supreme Court decision on elective abortion on disposition of premarital pregnancies. In 1971, when their first survey was conducted, most pregnancies ended in live births. This was far less common at the time of their second survey, in 1976. Variables positively related to abortion in 1976 included age, socioeconomic status, and age at first conception. Religiosity and wantedness of the pregnancy were positively related to live birth.

Another example of this approach was a longitudinal study by Evans et al. (1976), which looked at four groups of 13- to 19-year-olds (aborters, those who remained single and kept the child, those who married and kept the child, and those who thought they were pregnant but found out that they were not) both before and after the implementation of their pregnancy decisions. They examined such variables as socioeconomic background, school performance, religious and social activities, sources of financial support, attitudes toward contraception and abortion, knowledge about conception, and reasons that contraception was not used. Among their major findings were that those who kept their children tended to have school problems, while those who aborted did not, and that there was an increase in subjects' satisfaction with their pregnancy resolutions between the first and second interview.

A third, basically atheoretical, study was done by Fischman (1977), who studied never-married black urban adolescents between 13 and 18 experiencing their first pregnancies. Fischman found that those who kept their babies differed from aborters in having lower socioeconomic backgrounds, being more likely to be on welfare, not doing well in school, having longer and more stable relationships with their partners, having more satisfactory relations with their parents, and tending to be happy about their pregnancies. There is considerable agreement among atheoretical researchers in such findings, providing a cumulative descriptive base on which more theoretically oriented scholars can build.

In our examination of research using a more theoretical approach, three models will be used. The oldest, which was dominant prior to the legalization of elective abortion, is the deviance model, with a perspective of criminality, mental illness, pathology, or, at a minimum, inadequacy. In contrast to that is one that might be called the feminist model, although it generally has not been so titled by the researchers who have used it. This model is based on a perspective that women have a right to control their own bodies and that they exhibit competence and good coping skills in dealing with the resolution of their pregnancies. This resolution process typically is a learning experience for them. A recent model, which is more concerned with the decision-making process than the others, is a problem-solving model. Research may fall into several of these categories, of course. They are not necessarily mutually exclusive.

Deviance Model

Uncritical Application

This model often was applied uncritically to "unwanted" pregnancy before the legalization of elective abortion.[2] Sociologists, as well as social workers, focused mainly on "unwed motherhood" and "illegitimacy," which they saw as major social problems, and ignored the possibility of "unwanted" pregnancy among married women, as well as the pattern of marrying to legitimate a pregnancy. They frequently compared those who released their babies for adoption with those who kept their children (Jones et al., 1962: Meyer et al., 1959; Vincent, 1961). In designing their studies, they tended unquestioningly to accept the traditional role of women, in which the female was expected to find her supreme fulfillment in marriage and motherhood. Her sexual activity was defined as "normal" and acceptable only within a monogamous marriage relationship. Therefore, the fact of an "unwanted" pregnancy outside of marriage presupposed deviant sexual behavior.

A number of researchers working from this model indicated that there was something unique about the personality of single women that led them to choose to become unwed mothers (Malmquist et al., 1967; Meyerowitz and Malev, 1973; Otto, 1965; Schonholz et al, 1969). Young (1954), for instance, took the psychoanalytic position that such mothers were acting out deep conflicts and that they were passive, fearful, and had low self-esteem. Vincent (1961) found that respondents who kept their children had less positive results on the California Psychological Inventory than did either those who released their children for adoption or a sample of high school females tested by Gough (1960). He raised the question of whether these findings were measuring the psychosocial effects of an illicit pregnancy, rather than previously existing personality traits, but inexplicably concluded that the test scores could be interpreted as measuring primarily pre-pregnancy attitudes and behavior patterns. Meyer et al. (1959) concluded that there was a relationship between emotional maturity and giving the baby up for adoption rather than keeping it. It is interesting that earlier researchers (Rome, 1940; Bowlby, 1951) found just the contrary: Poor psychological functioning was considered to be characteristic of those who released their children for adoption rather than those who kept them. Obviously, the social climate was a significant factor in the conclusions presented. It should be noted that findings of a number of researchers were based on caseworkers' ratings of mental health done after the pregnancy resolution decision had been made, and may reflect primarily the caseworkers' opinions (Bowlby, 1951; Costigan, 1964; Meyer et al., 1956; Rome, 1940). More recent research has not tended to compare women who released their children for adoption with those who have kept their children, largely because such a small minority of women have chosen to release their child for adoption since the legalization of elective abortion. For instance, in my Michigan statewide study of pregnancy resolution, for which data were collected during 1974-1975, only 87 of 1,746 respondents chose to release their children for adoption (Rosen et al., 1976). It should be noted that subjects were obtained from maternity homes and so-called adoption agencies as well as numerous other sources.

Many researchers, uncritically accepting the deviance model, also have sought a relationship between the pregnant women's family relations (broken homes, parental absence, troubled families, relations with the mother) and the pregnancy resolution. They have expected and tended to find family pathology among those who keep their children (Daniels, 1969; Elster et al., 1980; Meyer et al, 1959; Youngs and Niebyl, 1975). For instance, Vincent (1961) found that those who kept their children more often came from unhappy and *mother-dominated* homes and lacked parental affection than did those who released their children for adoption.[3] Loesch and Greenberg (1962), who compared a group of single pregnant women in a maternity home, most of whom released their children for adoption, with a group of married pregnant women, provide another example of this perspective. They found that the unwed women showed more severe disturbance than did the married women, ignoring the fact that being, single, pregnant, and in a maternity home might be a very stressful experience. They indicated that the single women had had earlier experience with death, separation, and divorce and tended to have dependent relationships with others.

There have been a number of good critiques of studies that look for psychological causes of the "choice" of unmarried motherhood (Chilman, 1978; Furstenberg, 1976; Pauker, 1971; Rains, 1971). Chilman, for instance, has noted that many of these studies made the sexist assumption that only the woman who gives birth is responsible for the pregnancy, ignoring the father's role. Furstenberg (1976: 38) pointed out that researchers who assume that unwed motherhood springs from a special motivation ignore the fact that "to become an unwed mother, a woman must 'successfully' negotiate the entire course," and ignore those who marry before delivery, have an abortion, are not fecund, or have a "close call."

Most behavioral scientists who studied pregnancy resolution prior to the late 1960s, when the first states repealed restrictive abortion laws, did not attempt to consider the alternative to abortion, because of the difficulty of gaining access to women who chose that route. Abortion, whether illegal or therapeutic, was stigmatized and, consequently, secrecy was of the essence. Those women who were able to arrange for therapeutic abortions had to present themselves as mentally unstable or mentally ill, which was stigmatizing in itself, without the fact of "deviant" sexual behavior even being considered. This does not mean that no studies of therapeutic abortion were being carried out, however. The psychiatrists who were the gatekeepers for therapeutic abortion frequently studied their patients and tended to generalize from them to abortion seekers in general (Deutsch, 1945; Bolter, 1962; Fleck, 1970; Galdston, 1958). They ignored the large but elusive population of women who had illegal abortions or aborted themselves.

Psychiatrists continued to study abortion patients following the easing of restrictions on elective abortion. Behavioral scientists also began to study abortion seekers, turning away from unwed motherhood. Changes in the legal status of abortion did not prevent researchers from continuing uncritically to apply a deviant model to its study, however. The deviance of premarital sexual behavior was compounded for those who openly chose legal abortion by their refusal to pay the price of motherhoood for their "sins." Psychiatrists and some behavioral scientists continued to see women who made that choice as immature and sick, as having unconscious conflicts over their feminine identity, and/or as impulsive, acting out, anxious, and denying, with weak ego development and masochistic and aggressive tendencies (Downs and Clayson, 1972; Ford et al., 1972; Kane et al., 1973; Martin, 1973; Walbert and Butler, 1973). They saw women who sought abortions as having a traditional view of women's roles, in spite of their inability to accept motherhood, and as behaving in a manner considered characteristic of women — that is, acting passively, irrationally, illogically, and incompetently. As Emily Moore-Cavar (1974) has pointed out, the women seeking abortion — rather than their partners, the method, or the medical care system — were assumed to have failed. They were seen as emotionally disturbed exaggerations of the stereotype of women generally: immature in terms of the male definition of adult maturity as indicated by such social scientists as Broverman et al. (1970).

Among those uncritically using the deviance model, women who got abortions also commonly were seen as generally experiencing conflict over their decision, feeling guilt, shame, and ambivalence (Dauber et al., 1972; Kane and Lachenbruch, 1973; Pakter et al., 1973), although other studies have consistently refuted such findings (Evans et al, 1976; Fingerer, 1973; Osofsky and Osofsky, 1972; Perez-Reyes and Falk, 1973).

Some sociologists whose area of specialization is deviance, but who have had only peripheral interest in fertility behaviors, have included abortion in their texts even after legalization of elective abortion. For instance, Dinitz et al. (1975), in a section on abortion, discussed it in a context of "offenses and deviations without 'victims,' " along with prostitution and pornography. The authors defined the legalization of elective abortion as "decriminalization" of victimless acts. A sociologist such as Reiss (1970), who is known primarily for his work on sexuality, also grouped abortion, illegitimacy, prostitution, and premarital sexual activity as deviant. Other scholars have been concerned about the "problem" of abortion "recidivism" — a term with connotations of criminality and a relapse into negative behavior (Ram et al., 1974; Rovinsky, 1972).[4] By implication, these scholars are indicating negative qualities in those who chose abortion. Other deviance specialists, however, have been more objective. Davis (1975: 51), for instance, noted that "those that rank sexual equality and female autonomy as lesser values than the life of the human fetus tend to define abortion as dangerous deviance, while those with the opposite priority do not."

Critical Application

Another series of fertility behavior researchers have used the deviance model more critically and objectively, analyzing the feelings of the actors that their behaviors (sexual activity, pregnancy, and pregnancy resolution) have been deviant or morally reprehensible, or examining the impact of the stigmatization by society of such behaviors on the actors (Briedis, 1975; Rains, 1971; Rosen and Martindale, 1980; Ryan, 1971; Zimmerman, 1977). Rains, for instance, critically examined why unwed motherhood was seen as a social problem. She pointed out the fact that it often was falsely equated with illegitimate pregnancy, although most such pregnancies are resolved by marriage, abortion, or, if neither of those solutions is feasible, adoption. She indicated that her subjects perceived their premarital sexuality as deviant, needing neutralization through love and the expectation of marriage. Those who kept their children were not seen by her as freely making that choice, in most cases, but as having fewer alternatives available to them than those taking other routes. Zimmerman (1977: 63), in her study of abortion patients, found that her subjects perceived abortion as "something belonging to an underground, deviant side of society . . . something unsafe, unclean — even sinister," and believed that their fellow citizens also disapproved of abortion.

On the other hand, Rosen and Martindale (1980) indicated that while many researchers uncritically regarded legal elective abortion as "deviant," the subjects who had early abortions did not tend to view their actions in that light.

Browner (1975) explored the widely held assumption that abortion necessarily is a life crisis and trauma for those who undergo it, and found that more than half of her subjects fell into a noncrisis category and expressed no doubts or ambivalence about having the abortion.

Feminist Model

In this model, marriage and motherhood are not denigrated, but neither are they viewed as woman's sine qua non. If chosen, marriage and/or motherhood may legitimately be combined with career and other interests. Such personal characteristics as intelligence, competence, and self-determination are viewed as human, not simply male, qualities. Woman's sexuality is accepted and affirmed. Single parenthood or abortion are viewed as legitimate options. Feminists want to help women free themselves from traditional norms sufficiently so that they can accept at an emotional level their rights to control their own bodies and comfortably reject, at any given time and for any period of time, either a maternal, life-nurturing role or marriage inextricably tied to birth of a child. This model was used by activists promoting social change from the mid 1960s on, but was not utilized in research until after legalization of abortion.

As noted earlier, scholars who used this model did not label it. Most of them applied it in a critical way, as well, rather than simply basing their research on a set of "feminist" assumptions. By and large, they focused particularly on abortion. As David et al. (1978: 85) pointed out:

> Another psychological model, shared by Steinhoff (1977), Miller (1977) and TFRI (Transnational Family Research Institute), views abortion-seeking behavior as an effective means of coping with a personal crisis, a normal ego-enhancing development, more likely to have positive than negative psychological consequences. For example, in comparing aborting women with those who carried an unplanned pregnancy to term, whether in or out of wedlock, Steinhoff et al (1972) found that abortion patients were more future and planning oriented, had higher personal aspirations, and were more idealistic about marriage and eventual motherhood. Successful crisis resolution becomes a learning experience.

In my statewide Michigan study, I hypothesized that choice of abortion would be negatively associated with traditional attitudes toward the female role and positively associated with perceived competence. The basis for these hypotheses was explained as follows (Rosen et al., 1979: 121-122):

> A decision to abort indicate(s) activism rather than passivity. . . . It was reasoned that among the forces resulting in activism, in the

sense of willingness to commit oneself to a course of action, are a sense of competency/efficacy in coping with problems and a manifest concern for one's own rights. . . . Conformity to traditionally feminine qualities of dependence and passivity also should lead to non-action. . . . A woman's concern for her own rights today, on the other hand, often may take the form of an untraditional role orientation.

The hypothesis that choice of abortion would be negatively associated with traditional attitudes toward the female role was supported, but the hypothesis that choice of abortion would be positively associated with perceived competence was not borne out statistically, although the relationship was in the expected direction.

Freeman (1977, 1978) hypothesized that women who chose abortion would perceive themselves as agents — that is, as persons who would act on events in their lives. She stated (1977: 510) that "to choose abortion is a vigorous intervention in one's life, to deny passive acceptance of an unwanted pregnancy." She did not find clear support for this hypothesis, however. Rather, she found that most women chose abortion because of impersonal pressures on them. The decision and experience tended to be a learning experience, however, which resulted in increased self-management.

Some psychiatrists even tended toward this model, finding that dealing with pregnancy helped to develop new adaptive skills (Bibring and Valenstein, 1976). Also, Miller (1980) tentatively concluded from his longitudinal study of over 1,000 women, two-thirds of whom were married, that women who chose abortion rather than delivery were able to do so because of independence of mind and an assertiveness that helped them work through the emotionally difficult decision and then implement it.

Problem-Solving Model

In recent years, a number of researchers have looked at pregnancy resolution in terms of problem-solving abilities and processes. While several different theories are subsumed under the general heading, all assume that choices are determined, in part at least, by individuals' beliefs about the consequences of each alternative: the advantages compared to the disadvantages (see Bracken et al, 1978; Rosen, 1976; Steinhoff et al, 1971).

The importance of taking cognitive and moral development, as they relate to problem-solving abilities, into consideration in order to understand pregnancy resolutions has been stressed by several writers (Chilman, 1978; McKenry et al., 1979), but only rarely actually has been done. One interesting study (Gilligan, 1977) focused on an alternative for Kohlberg's stage theory of moral development that would apply more accurately to women than his model. Gilligan derived a three-stage alternative sequence from her research on women making a pregnancy resolution decision. Cobliner (1974), using Piaget's concepts, interpreted data obtained from various groups of adolescents as indicating figurative, rather than operative, thought. Hatcher (1976) also took a developmental approach in trying to understand adolescent pregnancy decisions and concluded that cognitive skills and logical thought were at their peak in late adolescence.

One of the earliest efforts to use a problem-solving approach to understanding fertility decisions was that of the Hawaii project researchers (Diamond et al., 1973; Steinhoff et al., 1971). The relationship of decisions concerning coitus, birth control, and pregnancy outcomes were posited, primarily in terms of how decisions concerning contraception affected pregnancy resolution decisions and how pregnancy resolution decisions then affected later decisions regarding contraception. Steinhoff (1978) also considered preferred choices and alternatives for pregnancy resolution, finding that marriage to legitimate the child was the option considered most often but also rejected most frequently. Most of those who did marry before delivery did not consider any other options, however.

Prominent among those working on decision-making models relevant to fertility behaviors has been Hollerbach (1978; Hass, 1974). Her model covers the whole range of decisions, from a cross-cultural perspective, including such postnatal choices as infanticide and abandonment, as well as the more commonly perceived choices of giving up a child for adoption or "lending" it to others to care for temporarily. Her focus has tended to be on married couples, but it can be applied to single individuals or nonmarital partners as well. Shedlin and Hollerbach (1981) applied her model to a rural Mexican community in 1975. They focused, however, on the preconception stage of decision-making, because information about pregnancy resolution was hampered by secrecy concerning abortion and infanticide. As far as they could ascertain, abortion was never discussed between spouses. She has also looked at how power and communication in families has affected fertility decision-making. Like Rosen et al. (1979), she has contrasted passive decision-making, or the implicit decision to do nothing, with active decision-making. Smetana and Adler (1979) also have used a problem-solving approach to a consideration of abortion. They analyzed pregnancy resolution decisions in terms of Fishbein's expectancy X value model of behavioral intention and found that the model was applicable to such choice situations. They went beyond Fishbein's model, however, to examine determinants of intention, finding that social-normative beliefs were particularly important. The role of beliefs in pregnancy resolution decisions was expanded by Smetana in other work (1979).

While Miller's work (1980) has concentrated on the decision of married couples to conceive intentionally, rather than on pregnancy resolution choice when a conception was not intended, he has developed a decision-making model that he applies to abortion as well as to the decisions to have children, to marry, or to separate. His model includes stages of decision-making and six psychological components of decision-making that occur at the various stages.

Bracken et al. (1978) used the Janis-Mann (1977) decision-making framework in their analyses, but quite superficially. Their data collection did not seem to have been structured in terms of the decision-making model, and their findings were not integrally tied to the model, although they developed a path analysis of the principal components of the decision to abort or deliver in terms of the model.

In my current research on pregnancy resolution among adolescents, a heuristic model, influenced by the work of Goldfried and Davison (1976), has been developed. My model includes eight steps: (1) the development of contingency plans concerning a possible problem — thinking ahead; (2) verification that a problem exists, which includes definition of a situation as problematical; (3) generation, consideration, and evaluation (alone or with others) of perceived alternative resolutions, which includes weighing the perceived rewards and costs of each alternative, either implicitly or explicitly; (4) choice of an alternative; (5) evaluation of the immediate consequences of one's choice on self and others; (6) change of the resolution decision in some cases; (7) implementation of the decision; and (8) evaluation of the consequences of one's actions after the decision has been implemented. This model was basic to the development of the interview schedules, as well as a critical guide for the analysis of data. The evaluation of alternatives, which is part of step 3, has been postulated to be based in part on the consequences of previous pregnancy resolution decisions; the role of significant others in the decision-making, including their definition of the situation and the extent and nature of their power in relation to the subject; and the subjects' aspirations, attitudes, and self-concept.

METHODOLOGICAL APPROACHES

Many of the methodological shortcoming of research in this area have been fairly consistent, regardless of theoretical perspective, and the relatively few well-designed and well-executed studies have not fallen into any one theoretical category.

Sampling

Overwhelmingly, the samples used in most pregnancy resolution research were small, biased convenience samples and of females only (with respect to male samples, see Chapter 4). Regarding sample size, for instance, Blumenfield (1978) used 26 patients from an outpatient abortion clinic, Hatcher (1973, 1976) had a sample of only 13 patients, Gilligan (1977) studied 29 women, and Schaffer and Pine (1972) used a sample of 24 girls at a New York City hospital prior to their abortions. Browner's (1975) sample was 22 women. Maternity home patients frequently were used as representative of women who delivered, because access to them was relatively convenient (Butts and Sporakowski, 1974; Kane and Lachenbruch, 1973; Loesch and Greenberg, 1962). Maternity home patients, however, are a very atypical group, and one cannot legitimately generalize from them to women who choose to bear their children. I found, for instance, that maternity home subjects were significantly more influenced by their mothers and had significantly more conflict over their decisions than did other women who bore their children (Rosen, 1976).

A frequent criticism is the lack of comparison or control groups in this research, and it is true that it has been common for scholars to use subjects from only one choice category and often only from a single clinic (Browner, 1975; Bracken and Kasl, 1975; Cobliner, 1974; Rosenthal and Rothchild, 1975; Shaw et al., 1979). Even among the considerable number who did use comparison groups, however, most studied clinic populations (Bracken et al, 1978; Fischman, 1977; Graves, 1975). This is understandable, since it is extremely difficult to obtain a random sample of individual women who are pregnant, and it is especially hard to identify and reach patients of private physicians. Because all abortions in Hawaii must be performed in hospitals, the Hawaii study was able to reach a representative time sample of all maternity and abortion patients in the state. This is a very unusual situation, however. As noted, Kantner and Zelnick carried out two national probability surveys of American teenagers (Zelnick et al., 1980; Zelnick and Kantner, 1974), in which they obtained retrospective data about their subjects' pregnancies.

My research has been innovative in sampling procedures, although not free from some of the problems that are almost universally experienced by scholars studying pregnancy resolution. One of my studies, a statewide one of "problem" pregnancies (Rosen et al., 1979), used a two-stage stratified sampling design. Organizations that served the population of interest in dealing with their pregnancies were stratified on the basis of caseload size, type of service provided, and geographic location. They included hospitals and clinics that provided abortion procedures, social agencies, maternity homes, continuing education programs for pregnant teenagers, and prenatal clinics, all of which serve women who planned to bear their children. Second, all clients of a sampled organization who were served during a specified time period were included in the sample. Patients of private physicians who sought no organizational help in dealing with their pregnancies — who resigned themselves to having an unplanned child without getting counsel or who used the gray or black market for adoption — were left out, however. Also, the refusal rate of organizations that served women who delivered was higher than optimal. In an effort to overcome such problems, a more recent study was designed that aimed to study all adolescents who sought pregnancy services in a single rural county during a fourteen-month period. Since all pregnancy services in that county were offered by private physicians, access to the subjects was obtained through those private physicians. This study consequently reached a group that previously had been largely untapped, as well as the total population of appropriate subjects during a given time period. This study was important in terms of sampling not only because it reached patients of private physicians, but also because the population studied was a rural one. Almost all studies have been of urban populations, and we know little about the differences or similarities between rural and urban pregnancy resolution decision-making.

Definition of Population

Some scholars lacked a clear definition of their populations of interest, as well. For instance, Zongker (1977) and DeAmicis et al. (1981) equated pregnancy with motherhood, leaving out the possibility that pregnancy could eventuate in abortion or miscarriage.

The title of Zonker's article is "The Self Concept of Pregnant Adolescent Girls," but he dealt only with those who made the decision to keep and rear their children. He used a control group that was a random sample of high school students and assumed that they were never pregnant, ignoring the possibility that a number of them might have been pregnant but resolved their pregnancies through abortion.

Cross-Sectional Studies

Another shortcoming of most pregnancy resolution studies, noted by many (Chilman, 1978; Newman, 1973; Payne et al., 1973), has been their cross-sectional nature. If one is to understand process, longitudinal research is imperative. The problem of subject attrition is a serious one, however, for which no foolproof solutions have been found. For instance, my recent research aimed at three interviews for all subjects, one prior to implementation of the pregnancy resolution decision and two at six-week and six-month periods following implementation. Of the 100 subjects who responded to the first interview, however, only 36 completed the second interview and 31 participated in the third. This is a common phenomenon. Few explicitly refused to cooperate in the later interviews. More often the respondent failed to appear for appointments or could not be reached. A number had moved away and could not be located. As Adler (1976) points out, however, the attrition is not a problem in itself. If those who take part in the later interviews do not differ on critical variables from those who do not, there is no major problem. In my study, nonrespondents to the later interviews did not differ significantly from the respondents in terms of age, religion, relations with partner at conception, pregnancy resolution decision, or socioeconomic status.

While not directly focused on pregnancy resolution, Adler made a review of 17 studies, done between 1966 and 1973, in which subjects originally were contacted before their abortions and then again at some time afterwards. The percentages of the initial sample lost to follow-up ranged from a low of 13 percent to a high of 86 percent. A number of these researchers also found no significant differences between respondents to later interviews and nonrespondents, but Adler concluded that, in general, younger women and Catholic women were less likely to take part in follow-up, as well as women for whom the abortion was particularly stressful.

Other Problems

Quite a few studies of pregnancy resolution have been retrospect-ive, with all the recall distortion and reconstruction of reality in order to avoid cognitive dissonance to which such resarch is liable (see Chesney-Lind, 1979; Zimmerman, 1977). With retrospective re-search, also, one can not distinguish between effects produced by implementation of the decision and conditions that existed previ-ously. There also have been a number of prospective studies which, while they may have had other drawbacks, established a baseline before implementation of the pregnancy resolution decision and then measured the later impact of the decision (see Evans et al., 1976; Graves, 1975; Hatcher, 1973, 1976). Even the prospective studies have limitations, however; the baseline data may have been affected by the subjects' pregnancies.

Lack of comparability in instruments and tests used is another shortcoming of much research in this area. While many studies have employed standardized tests, few have used the same ones, with the exception of the Minnesota Multiphasic Personality Inventory and Rotter's Locus of Control scale.

SUMMARY

Since most studies of pregnancy resolution decison-making, as a process, have occurred within the last ten years, one would not expect all the kinks in such research to be ironed out by now. The very fact that attention has become focused on the process rather than on correlates of choice is a major step forward, and many earlier value-laden assumptions about correlates have been disproved, leaving researchers freer to move ahead to new fields. To the extent that choices in favor of abortion and single parenthood become less stig-matized by society, it should be easier to follow up subjects over time. That is, they are likely to feel more open about their experiences if they think that their actions are accepted. There is considerable agreement on goals, such as the importance of longitudinal research, in-depth collection of data, and use of comparable instruments, and that, in and of itself, should be a useful spur to future researchers.

NOTES

1. One other pssible pregnancy resolution is suicide, but this alternative has been studied rarely. One study that did examine suicide among pregnant teenagers was done by Gabrielson et al. (1970). It was not clear whether suicide attempts by this group were a pregnancy resolution choice, however, or whether both the pregnancy and the suicide attempt were consequences of disturbance on the part of the subjects. Otto (1965) also reported on suicide attempts by pregnant women under the age of 21.

2. It was generally assumed that all unanticipated pregnancies of single women were unwanted, while all pregnancies of married women, planned or not, were wanted. In recent years, researchers have examined critically the concepts of "wantedness" and "unwantedness." See for instance, Hass (1974) and Miller (1974).

3. Vincent (1961: 118) was contradictory in his interpretation of findings. For instance, with respect to the concept of "mother dominated homes," in an earlier chapter he noted the probability " that the majority of females in the United States come from homes dominated by one person — usually the mother." In the later chapter, he felt the difference between those who kept their children and those who released them for adoption was a very important one, which he put in italics. He strove to be objective and scientific in his analyses, but he often got trapped in the values of his time.

4. It is interesting that the term "recidivism" also has been used for multiparae (Bowerman et al., 1966). Emily Moore-Cavar (1974: 365) was mistaken when she said, " It seems doubtful that the term would be used in reference to women who have had more than one unplanned birth. "

REFERENCES

Adler, N. E. Sample attrition in studies of psychosocial sequelae of abortion: How great a problem? *Journal of Applied Social Psychology,* 1976, 6(3), 240-259.

Bibring, G. L., and Valenstein, A. F. Psychological aspects of pregnancy. *Clinical Obstetrics and Gynecology,* 1976, 19, 357-371.

Blumenfield, M. Psychological factors involved in request for elective abortion. *Journal of Clinical Psychiatry.* 1978, 39, (January), 17-25.

Bolter, S. The psychiatrist's role in therapeutic abortion: The unwitting accomplice. *American Journal of Psychiatry,* 1962, 119, (October), 312-316.

Bowerman, C., Irish, D., and Pope, H. *Unwed motherhood: Personal and social consequences.* Chapel Hill: University of North Carolina Institute for Research in Social Science, 1966.

Bowlby, J. *Maternal care and mental health.* Geneva: World Health Organization, 1951.

Bracken, M. B., and Kasl, S. V. Delay in seeking induced abortion: A review and theoretical analysis. *American Journal of Obstetrics and Gynecology,* 1975, 121(7), 1008-1019.

Bracken, M. B., Klerman, L. V., and Bracken, M. Coping with pregnancy resolution among never-married women. *American Journal of Orthopsychiatry,* 1978, 48(2), 320-334. (a)

Bracken, M. B., Klerman, L. V., and Bracken, M. Abortion, adoption, or mother-hood: An empirical study of decision-making during pregnancy. *American Journal of Obstetrics and Gynecology,* 1978, 130(3), 251-262. (b)

Briedis, C. Mariginal deviants: Teenage girls experience community response to premarital sex and pregnancy. *Social Problems,* 1975, 22(4), 480-493.

Broverman, I. K., Broverman, D. B., Carlson, F., Rosenkrantz, P., and Vogel, S. Sex-role stereotypes and clinical judgments of mental health. *Journal of Consulting and Clinical Psychology,* 1970, 34(1), 1-7.

Browner, C. *Abortion as a life crisis.* 1975. (Mimeo; see *The Papers of the Kroeber Anthropological Society,* 1975, 47)

Butts, R. Y., and Sporakowski, M. J. Unwed pregnancy decisions: Some background factors. *Journal of Sex Research,* 1974, 10(2), 110-117.

Chesney-Lind, M. *Protest motherhood: Pregnancy decision-making behavior and attitudes toward abortion.* Paper presented at the annual meeting of the American Sociological Association, August 1979, Boston.

Chilman, C. S. *Adolescent sexuality in a changing American society: Social and psychological perspectives.* Washington, DC: Government Printing Office, 1978.

Cobliner, W. G. Pregnancy in the single adolescent girl: The role of cognitive functions. *Journal of Youth and Adolescence,* 1974, 3(1), 17-29.

Costigan, B. *The unmarried mother – Her decision regarding adoption.* D.S.W. thesis, University of Southern California, 1964. (Cited in S. MacIntyre, *Single and Pregnant.* New York: Prodist, 1977.)

Cushner, I. M., Oppel, W. C., Unger, H. T., Athansiou, R. B., and Yager, M. J. The Johns Hopkins experience. In H. Osofsky and J. Osofsky (Eds.), *The abortion experience.* New York: Harper & Row, 1973, 135-164.

Daniels, A. M. Reaching unwed mothers. *American Journal of Nursing,* 1969, 69, 332-335.

Dauber, B., Zalar, M., and Goldstein, P. J. Abortion counseling and behavioral change. *Family Planning Perspectives,* 1972, 4 (April), 23-27.

David, H. P., Friedman, H. L., van der Tak, J., and Sevilla, M. J. (Eds.). *Abortion in psychosocial perspective: Trends in transnational research.* New York: Springer, 1978.

Davis, F. J. Beliefs, values, power and public definitions of deviance. In F. J. Davis and R. Stivers (Eds.), *The collective definition of deviance.* New York: Free Press, 1975, 50-72.

De Amicis, L. A., Korman, R., Hess, D. W., and Mc Anarney, E. R. A comparison of unwed pregnant teenagers and nulligravid sexually active adolescents seeking contraception. *Adolescence,* 1981, 16, 11-20.

Deutsch, H. *Psychology of women: A psychoanalytic interpretation.* New York: Grune & Stratton, 1945.

Diamond, M., Steinhoff, P. G., Palmore, J. A., and Smith, R. G. Sexuality, birth control and abortion: A decision-making sequence. *Journal of Biosocial Science,* 1973, 5, 347-361.

Dinitz, S., Dynes, R. R., and Clarke, A. C. *Deviance: Studies in definition, management and treatment* (2nd ed.). New York: Oxford University Press, 1975.

Downs, L. A., and Clayson, D. *Unwanted pregnancy: A clinical syndrome defined by the similarities of preceding stressful events in the lives of women with particular personality characteristics.* Paper presented at the meeting of the American College of Obstetricians and Gynecologists, 1972.

Elster, A. B., Panzarine, S., and Mc Anarney, E. R. Causes of adolescent pregnancy. *Medical Aspects of Human Sexuality,* 1980, 14, 69-87.

Evans, J., Selstad, G., and Welcher, W. Teenagers: Fertility control behavior and attitudes before and after abortion, childbearing or negative pregnancy test. *Family Planning Perspectives,* 1976, 8(4), 192-200.

Fingerer, M. Psychological sequelae of abortion: Anxiety and depression. *Journal of Community Psychology,* 1973, 1, 221-225.

Fischman, S. Delivery or abortion in inner-city adolescents. *American Journal of Orthopsychiatry,* 1977, 47(1), 127-133.

Fleck, S. Some psychiatric aspects of abortion. *Journal of Nervous and Mental Disease,* 1970, 151, 42-50.

Ford, C. V., Castelnuovo-Tedesco, P., and Long, K. D. Women who seek therapeutic abortion: A comparison study with women who complete their pregnancy. *American Journal of Psychiatry,* 1972, 129 (December), 546-552.

Freeman, E. W. Influence of personality attributes on abortion experiences. *American Journal of Orthopsychiatry,* 1977, 47(3), 503-513.

Freeman, E. W. Abortion: Subjective attitudes and feelings. *Family Planning Perspectives,* 1978, 10(3), 150.

Furstenberg, F. F., Jr. *Unplanned parenthood.* New York: Free Press, 1976.

Gabrielson, I. W., Klerman, L. V., Currie, J. B., Tyler, N. C., and Jekel, J. F. Suicide attempts in a population pregnant as teenagers. *American Journal of Public Health,* 1970, 60, 2289-2301.

Galdston, I. In M. E. Calderone (Ed.), *Abortion in the United States.* New York: Harper & Row, 1958.

Gilligan, C. In a different voice: Women's conceptions of self and morality. *Harvard Educational Review,* 1977, 47, 481-517.

Goldfried, M., and Davison, G. C. *Clinical Behavior Therapy.* New York: Holt, Rinehart, & Winston, 1976.

Gough, H. G. Theory and measurement of socialization. *Journal of Consulting Psychology,* 1960, 24, 23-30.

Graves, W. L. Sequelae of unwanted pregnacy: A comparison of unmarried abortion and maternity patients. Unpublished Manuscript, Department of Gynecology and Obstetrics, Emory University School of Medicine, Atlanta, Georgia, 1975.

Hass, P. H. Wanted and unwanted pregnancies: A fertility decision-making model. *Journal of Social Issues,* 1974, 30, 125-165.

Hatcher, S. L. The adolescent experience of pregnancy and abortion: A developmental analysis. *Journal of Youth and Adolescence,* 1973, 2(1), 53-102.

Hatcher, S. L. Understanding adolescent pregnancy and abortion. *Primary Care,* 1976, 3(3), 407-424.

Hollerbach, P. E. New directions in psychosocial models of fertility decision making. *Population and Environmental Psychology Newsletter,* 1978, 5(1), 14-19.

Janis, I. L., and Mann, L. *Decision-making: A psychological analysis of conflict, choice and commitment.* New York: Free Press, 1977.

Jones, W. C., Meyer, H. F., and Borgatta, E. F. Social and psychological factors in status decision of unmarried mothers. *Marriage and Family Living,* 1962, 24 (August), 224-230.

Kane, F. J., and Lachenbruch, P. A. Adolescent pregnancy: A study of aborters and non-aborters. *American Journal of Orthopsychiatry,* 1973, 43(5), 796-803.

Kane, F. J., Jr., Lachenbruch, P., Lipton, M., and Baram, D. Motivational factors in abortion patients. *American Journal of Psychiatry,* 1973, 130 (March), 290-293.

Loesch, J. G., and Greenberg, N. A. Some specific areas of conflicts observed during pregnancy. *American Journal of Orthopsychiatry,* 1962, 32, 624-636.

Macintyre, S. *Single and pregnant.* London: Croom Helm, 1977.

Malmquist, C. P., Kiresuk, T., and Spano, R. Mothers with multiple illegitimacies. *Psychiatric Quarterly,* 1967, 339-354.

Martin, C. Psychological problems of abortion for the unwed teenage girl. *Genetic Psychiatric Monograph*, 1973, 88, 23-110.

McKenry, P. C., Walters, L. H., and Johnson, C. Adolescent pregnancy: A review of the literature. *The Family Coordinator*, January 1979, 17-28.

Meyer, H. J., Borgatta, E. F., and Fanshel, D. Unwed mothers' decisions about their babies: An interim replication study. *Child Welfare*, 1959, 38 (February), 1-6.

Meyer, H. J., Jones, W., and Borgatta E. F. The decision of unmarried mothers to keep or surrender their babies. *Social Work*, 1956, 1 (April), 103-109.

Meyerowitz, J. H., and Malev, J. S. Pubescent attitudinal correlates antecedent to adolescent illegitimate pregnancy. *Journal of Youth and Adolescence*, 1973, 2(3), 251-258.

Miller, W. Relationships between the intendedness of conception and wantedness of pregnancy. *Journal of Nervous and Mental Disease*, 1974, 59, 396-406.

Miller, W. B. *The Psychology of reproduction.* Final report to the Center for Population Research, NICHD (NOI-HD-82831) by the American Institutes for Research, Palo Alto, California, 1980.

Moore-Cavar, E. C. *International inventory of information on induced abortion.* New York: Columbia University International Institute for the Study of Human Reproduction, 1974.

Newman S. H. Abortion: Needed behavioral-social research. In H. J. Osofsky and J. D. Osofsky (Eds.), *The abortion experience.* New York: Harper & Row, 1973.

Osofsky, J., and Osofsky, H. The psychological reaction of patients to legalized abortions. *American Journal of Orthopsychiatry*, 1972, 42, 48-60.

Otto, U. Suicidal attempts made by pregnant women under 21 years. *Acta Paedopsychiatry*, 1965, 32, 276-288.

Pakter, J., O'Hare, D., Nelson, F., and Svigir, M. A review of two years' experience in New York City with the liberalized abortion law. In H. J. Osofsky and J. D. Osofsky (Eds.), *The abortion experience.* New York: Harper & Row, 1973, 47-93.

Pauker, J. Girls pregnant out of wedlock. *Journal of Operational Psychiatry*, 1971, 1, 15-19.

Payne, E. C., Anderson, J. V., Kravitz, A. R., and Notman, M. T. Methodological issues in therapeutic abortion research. In H. J. Osofsky and J. D. Osofsky (Eds.), *The abortion experience.* New York: Harper & Row, 1973, 261-279.

Perez-Reyes, M. G., and Falk, R. Follow-up after therapeutic abortion in early adolescence. *Archives of General Psychiatry*, 1973, 28, 120-126.

Rains, P. *Becoming an unwed mother.* Chicago: Aldine, 1971.

Ram, B., Aguirre, B. E., and Wong, H-W. *Contraception and abortion recidivism.* Paper presented at the North Central Sociological Association Annual Meeting, Columbus, Ohio, May 1, 1974.

Reiss, I. L. Premarital sex as deviant behavior: An application of current approaches to deviance. *American Sociological Review*, 1970, 35, 78-87.

Rome, R. A method of predicting the probable disposition of their children by unmarried mothers. *Smith College Studies in Social Work*, 1940, 10, 167-201.

Rosen, R. H. Decision making on unplanned problem pregnancies. Final report to NICHD (HDO7739), 1976. (Mimeo)

Rosen, R. H., Ager, J. W., and Martindale, L. J. Contraception, abortion and self concept. *Journal of Population*, 1979, 2(2), 118-139.

Rosen, R. H., and Martindale, L. J. Abortion as "deviance": Traditional female roles vs. the feminist perspective. *Social Psychiatry*, 1980, 15, 103-108.

Rosen, R. H., Martindale, L. J., and Grisdela, M. *Pregnancy study report.* Detroit: Wayne State University, 1976. (Mimeo)

Rosenthal, M. B., and Rothchild, E. Some psychological considerations in adolescent pregnancy and abortion. *Advances in Planned Parenthood,* 1975, 9(3/4), 60-69.

Rovinsky, J. J. Abortion recidivism: A problem in preventive medicine. *Obstetrics and Gynecology,* 1972, 39, 649-659.

Ryan, W. *Blaming the victim.* New York: Vintage, 1971.

Schaffer, C., and Pine, F. Pregnancy, abortion, and the developmental tasks of adolescence. *American Academy of Child Psychiatry Journal,* 1972, 11, 511-536.

Schonholz, D. H., Gusberg, S. B., Astrachan, J. M., Davidson, A. B., Morganthau, J., Young, A. T., Gouley, C., Simon, B., and Cox, L. An adolescent guidance program: Study in education for marital health. *Obstetrics and Gynecology,* 1969, 34, 610-614.

Shaw, P. C., Funderburk, C., and Franklin, B. J. Investigation of the abortion decision process. *Psychology, a Quarterly Journal of Human Behavior,* 1979, 16(2), 11-19.

Shedlin, M. G., and Hollerbach, P. E. Modern and traditional fertility regulation in a Mexican community. *Studies in Family Planning,* 1981, 12, 278-296.

Smetana, J. G. Beliefs about the permissibility of abortion and their relationship to decision regarding abortion. *Journal of Population,* 1979, 2(4), 294-305.

Smetana, J. G., and Adler, N. E. Decision-making regarding abortion: A value x expectancy analysis. *Journal of Population,* 1979, 2, 338-357.

Steinhoff, P. G. Premarital pregnancy and the first birth. In W. B. Miller and L. F. Newman (Eds.), *The first child and family formation.* Chapel Hill, NC: Carolina Population Center, 1978, 180-208.

Steinhoff, P. G., Smith, R. G., and Diamond, M. The Hawaii pregnancy, birth control, and abortion study: Social-psychological aspects. In *Conference proceedings: Psychological measurement in the study of population problems.* Berkeley: University of California Institute of Personality Assessment and Research, 1971.

Vincent, C. E. *Unmarried mothers.* New York: Free Press, 1961.

Walbert, D., and Butler, D. *Abortion, society, and the law.* Cleveland: Case Western Reserve University Press, 1973.

Young, L. *Out of wedlock.* New York: McGraw-Hill, 1954.

Youngs, D. D., and Niebyl, J. R. Adolescent pregnancy and abortion. *Medical Clinics of North America,* 1975, 59(6), 1419-1427.

Zelnick, M., and Kantner, J. F. The resolution of teen-age first pregnancies. *Family Planning Perspectives,* 1974, 6(2), 74-80.

Zelnick, M., Kantner, J. F., and Ford, K. Adolescent pathways to pregnancy. Final report to NICHD, 1981. (Contract NOI-HD-82848)

Zimmerman, M. K. *Passage through abortion: A sociological analysis.* New York: Praeger, 1977.

Zongker, C. E. The self concept of pregnant adolescent girls. *Adolescence,* 1977, 12(48), 477-488.

The Contributors

LEE ROY BEACH is currently Professor and Chair of the Department of Psychology at the University of Washington in Seattle. He has been interested for some time in decision-making and childbearing.

LINDA J. BECKMAN is an Adjunct Associate Professor of Psychiatry at the University of California, Los Angeles. She received her A.B. from the University of Michigan and her M.A. and Ph.D. from UCLA. Dr. Beckman's principal research and writings have involved the fields of alcoholism, sociological and psychological aspects of aging, and population issues including couples' decision-making processes regarding childbearing and the long-term effects of childlessness for the individual. She is interested not only in the application of psychological theory to these subjects, but also in the improvement of survey research methodology as it applies to these areas.

TWYLAH BENSON received her B.A. and M.A. from the University of Houston and her Ph.D. in sociology from Wayne State University in 1980. She is currently an Assistant Professor of Sociology at Thiel College in Greenville, Pennsylvania. Her research interests focus on the family and religion.

FREDERICK L. CAMPBELL is currently Professor and Chair of the Department of Sociology at the University of Washington in Seattle. He has a long-standing interest in fertility behavior, and he and his colleagues, Beach and Townes, have been collaborating on studies of childbearing decisions for several years.

CANDICE FEIRING is Coordinator of the Infant Laboratory at Rutgers Medical School — UMDNJ. Research on family interaction and its relationship to the social and cognitive development of young children is a primary interest. She is also involved in the application of theory and research to evaluation and practice in community settings.

BRUCE R. FOX is currently a program consultant in agency relations at the United Foundation in Detroit, Michigan. He has taught sociology courses including sociology of sex roles at Wayne State University, the University of Vermont, and St. Michael's College. He received his Ph.D. in psychology with a specialization in social psychology from the University of Michigan in 1975.

GREER LITTON FOX is currently Professor of Sociology and Director of the Family Research Center at Wayne State University in Detroit, Michigan. She received her A.B. from Randolph-Macon Woman's College and her M.A. and Ph.D. from the University of Michigan. She was principal investigator for the study, "Mother-Daughter Communication Patterns re Sexuality," sponsored by the National Institute of Child and Human Development. In addition to her interests in intergenerational female socialization, she is engaged in research on the familial impacts of economic uncertainty.

DEBORAH I. FRANK, RN, Ph.D., is a sex therapist and educator certified by the American Association of Sex Educators, Counselors and Therapists. She also maintains a private clinical practice in sex therapy and is Clinical Instructor of Nursing at Florida State University, Tallahassee, Florida. She received her doctorate from the Interdivisional Program of Marriage and Family at Florida State University. Her previous publications and research deal with sexual adjustment after mastectomy and causal attributions of success and failure to attain orgasm.

KATHARINE A. FROHARDT-LANE received her A.B. from Oberlin College, her M.P.H. from the University of California at Berkeley, and her Ph.D. in population planning from the University of Michigan. Until recently she was a researcher/evaluator at a health maintenance organization in Detroit, Michigan. Currently she is a consultant to a national adult education consortium working with a project concerned with the socialization of educational aspirations.

Her major research interest is in the area of the effects of a birth on individual and family well-being.

FRANK F. FURSTENBERG, Jr., is Professor of Sociology at the University of Pennsylvania and author of *Unplanned Parenthood: The Social Consequences of Teenage Childbearing*. He is currently working on a longitudinal study of effects of marital disruption on children.

ROBERTA HERCEG-BARON is Coordinator of Research Activities at the Family Planning Council of Southeastern Pennsylvania. She is currently working on a project that involves interviewing a random sample of the mothers of the adolescents who participated in the study referred to here.

HELEN P. KOO is a Senior Demographer at Research Triangle Institute's Center for Population and Rural-Urban Studies, where she has worked since 1972, conducting research on adolescent fertility, childlessness, and the interrelationships among fertility, marital instability, and remarriage. Born in China, she received a B.A. in biological sciences from Stanford University and an M.S. in zoology from the University of Minnesota before going to the University of Nigeria to teach zoology. When the Nigerian civil war broke out in 1967, she returned home and decided to change her field to the study of human population dynamics. She therefore enrolled at the University of Michigan, receiving an M.P.H. and a Ph.D. degree in population planning.

MICHAEL LEWIS is Professor and Director of the Institute for the Study of Exceptional Children at Rutgers Medical School — UMDNJ. Dr. Lewis supervises a wide range of research activities that focus on social, cognitive, affective, and linguistic development in infancy and childhood in normal and handicapped children. He also holds a Clinical Professorship in Pediatric Psychology at the College of Physicians and Surgeons, Columbia University, New York.

ANN V. McGILLICUDDY-DeLISI is a Research Psychologist at Educational Testing Service. She received her Ph.D. from Catholic University in 1974. Her current interests include the role of the family as an influence on children's cognitive development.

RAYE HUDSON ROSEN is Professor of Sociology at Wayne State University, Detroit, Michigan. She obtained her M.A. from Columbia University and her Ph.D. from Yale, and has been involved in research dealing with social-psychological aspects of fertility for the last ten years. She was project director of a nationwide study of health professionals' attitudes concerning family planning and has been principal investigator of two studies of decision-making on pregnancy resolution.

JOHN SCANZONI is Professor of Child and Family Science and of Sociology at the University of North Carolina-Greensboro. Formerly, he was Professor of Sociology at Indiana University-Bloomington. His books include *Family Decision-Making; Sex Roles, Women's Work and Marital Conflict; The Black Family in Modern Society;* and *Sexual Bargaining.* His articles have appeared in *Journal of Marriage and Family,* and *American Sociological Review.* Continuing research interests center on the implications of changing gender roles for marriage, family and sexuality.

IRVING E. SIGEL is a Senior Research Psychologist at Educational Testing Service. He received his Ph.D. from the University of Chicago in 1951. After having been at Michigan State University, The Merrill-Palmer Institute, SUNY/Buffalo, he came to ETS in 1973 to embark on a research program in child development. His interests are in the social factors influencing cognitive development, particularly familial factors.

C. M. SUCHINDRAN is Associate Professor of Biostatistics, University of North Carolina at Chapel Hill. He received his M.Sc. in statistics from the University of Kerala, India, and his Ph.D. in biostatistics from the University of North Carolina at Chapel Hill. His primary research interests are in mathematical demography and statistical inference. His current research includes studies of interrelationships among marital disruptions, fertility, and remarriage; interrelationships between infant mortality and fertility; and computer simulation techniques for demographic analysis.

JAMES A. SWEET is Professor of Sociology at the University of Wisconsin — Madison, where he is affiliated with the Center for Demography and Ecology and the Institute for Research on Poverty.

He has published on the topics of the employment of married women, fertility trends, and divorce and remarriage. His recent research has focused on recent changes in the ways in which young women and men organize the major activities of the young adult years and on changing household and family patterns in the United States.

BRENDA D. TOWNES is Professor of Psychiatry and Behavioral Sciences at the University of Washington at Seattle. She joined the faculty in 1961 and has a strong interest in two areas: fertility decisions and clinical neuropsychology.

DATE DUE